Yang Style
Tai Ji Quan:
A Beginner's Guide

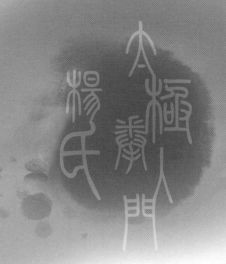

Project Editor: Mei Li & Liu Shui
Book & Cover Designer: Guo Miao
Typesetter: He Mei-ling

International Standard Library of Chinese Medicine

Yang Style
Tai Ji Quan:
A Beginner's Guide

Hu Zhen
Professor and Head of Department of Traditional Chinese Medicine
Wenzhou Medical College, Wenzhou, China

Xu Shi-zu
Chinese Traditional Sports and Health Cultivation Instructor,
School of Physical Education in Wenzhou Medical College, Wenzhou, China

Hon K. Lee
Director of the Jow Ga Shaolin Institute, Herndon, Virginia, USA

Li Wan-ling
Qi Gong and TCM Translator, Beijing, China

人民卫生出版社
PMPH PEOPLE'S MEDICAL PUBLISHING HOUSE

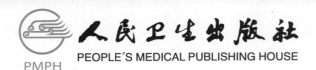

PEOPLE'S MEDICAL PUBLISHING HOUSE

PMPH

Website: http://www.pmph.com/en

Book Title: Yang Style Tai Ji Quan: A Beginner's Guide
(International Standard Library of Chinese Medicine)
太极拳入门：杨氏（国际标准化英文版中医教材）

Contact address: No. 19, Pan Jia Yuan Nan Li, Chaoyang District, Beijing 100021, P.R. China, phone/fax: 8610 5978 7338, E-mail: pmph@pmph.com

For text and trade sales, as well as review copy enquiries, please contact PMPH at pmphsales@gmail.com

First published: 2010
ISBN: 978-7-117-13353-1/R · 13354

Cataloguing in Publication Data:
A catalogue record for this book is available from the CIP-Database China.

ISBN 978-7-117-13353-1

9 787117 133531 >

Printed in The People's Republic of China

About the Authors

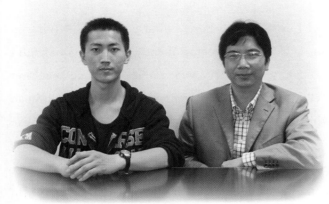

Hu Zhen (胡臻) & Xu Shi-zu (徐士祖)

Professor **Hu Zhen** is Dean of the School of International Education and head of the Department of Traditional Chinese Medicine at Wenzhou Medical College. He is a leading doctor of Traditional Chinese Medicine (TCM), one of Wenzhou's most renowned physicians, and one of the nation's most outstanding TCM clinicians.

Hu Zhen started to learn wu shu[1] from his father as a child, and later learned Yang style tai ji quan from Hu Guo-liang, who was a student of Master Zheng Man-qing. In 1992, Hu went to Brazil to be a visiting professor. In May 1995, he was the first to be appointed by the State Ministry of Health and the Health Bureau of Zhejiang Province as captain of the Chinese medical team to Namibia. While working in Namibia, he joined the medical team of the president's office at the invitation of President Nujoma. He was responsible for the medical care of the president and the first lady. He was also received warmly by Chairman Jiang Ze-min of China. In 2005, Hu went to Thailand and established a traditional Chinese medical center at Burapha University, and was the Chinese Dean of the Confucius Institute of Burapha University from 2007 to 2008.

Main works by Hu Zhen include: *The Chinese Doctor in the President's House* (总统府里的中国医生), *Clinical Reasoning of Chinese Medicine* (中医临证推理) - English Edition, *Chinese Medicine Tongue Diagnosis in Clinical Practice* (中医临床舌诊)-Chinese-Thai Bilingual Edition.

Xu Shi-zu graduated with a master's degree from Beijing Sports University, majored in traditional sports and concentrated on the study of sports and health cultivation. Xu participated in a demonstration of national research topics on the "Competition Routine of The Eight Pieces of Brocade," and "The Twelve Pieces of Brocade (Sitting Form)," and participated in composing a national research topic, "The Free Wandering Crane Elixir Routine." Xu is now a lecturer at the School of Physical Education in Wenzhou Medical College.

Xu started to learn wu shu from the age of 9, and inherited the *Hun Yuan* Internal Practice of the Wudang school from his family. He focused on the Wudang 128 Movements Tai Ji Quan Routine as well as Yang style tai ji quan. With a solid foundation in wu shu, Xu frequently participated in city or provincial teenage contests and achieved remarkable results. He earned a bachelor's degree with a wu shu major from the Hebei Institute of Physical Education. Xu focused on the practice of tai ji quan. Since then, he has visited and been guided by many tai ji quan masters.

---

[1] Wu shu is a generic term for both contemporary and traditional forms of Chinese martial arts.

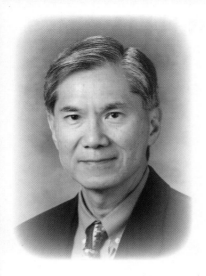

Hon K. Lee (李汉光)

Hon K. Lee is a U.S.-born Chinese American living in Washington, D.C. He is Director of the U.S. Jow Ga Shaolin Institute, and has over forty years of experience teaching traditional Chinese martial arts, including Yang style tai ji quan and Shaolin kung fu. He also practices traditional Chinese medicine, including qi gong therapy, and is owner of the Sports Edge Acupuncture Clinic.

As a child he learned martial arts basics from his uncle. In high school and college he practiced wrestling, judo, karate and taekwondo. He also studied with many well-known masters of Chen, Wu, and Yang style tai ji quan. He learned Jow Ga Kung Fu from Master Dean Chin and Master Chan Man-cheung, and Mizong Quan and Qingping Sword from Master Lu Jun-hai. He is a 3rd generation Jow Ga Kung Fu successor, a 7th generation Mizong Quan successor, and a 10th generation Qingping Sword successor.

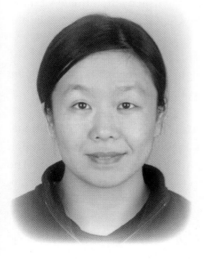

Li Wan-ling (Phoenix Li, 李云宁)

Li Wan-ling (a.k.a. Phoenix Li) was born in mainland China and moved to Hong Kong with her family as a child. She attended college in the United States and graduated with a bachelor's degree in business management in 1997. She received a second bachelor's degree in Traditional Chinese Medicine from Beijing University of Chinese Medicine (BUCM) in 2008. She is a Registered Chinese Medicine Practitioner in Hong Kong, and practices Traditional Chinese Medicine, including acupuncture and tui na therapy.

She has practiced qi gong and yoga for years, and since 2003 studied *Emei* (峨眉) *dǎo yǐn* and medicine with Master Zhang Ming-liang (张明亮), who is the lineage successor of master Zhou Qian-chuan (周潜川). She continues to study and extensively research TCM, qi gong, *dǎo yǐn*, Buddhism, Daoism, and many other areas of traditional Chinese culture.

Editorial Board for *International Standard Library of Chinese Medicine*

Russell William James, M.S. TCM
IELTS Examiner & Marker, *Beijing, China*

Jia De-xian (贾德贤)**, Ph.D. TCM**
Professor of Chinese Materia Medica, Beijing University of CM, Beijing, China

Jin Hong-zhu (金宏柱)
Professor of Acupuncture & Tui Na, Nanjing University of TCM, Nanjing, China

Lao Li-xing (劳力行)**, Ph.D.**
Professor of Acupuncture and Moxibustion, University of Maryland School of Medicine, Baltimore, USA Past Co-President of the Society for Acupuncture Research

Hon K. Lee (李汉光)**, Dipl. OM, L.Ac.**
Director of the Jow Ga Shaolin Institute, Herndon, Virginia, USA

Li Dao-fang (李道坊)**, Ph.D. TCM**
President of Florida Acupuncture Association; Executive Board Director, National Federation of Chinese TCM Organizations, Kissimmee, USA

Mei Li (李梅)**, M.S. TOM, L.Ac.**
Translator and Editor, People's Medical Publishing House, Beijing, China

Li Ming-dong (李名栋)**, Ph.D. OMD, L.Ac.**
Professor of Chinese Internal Medicine, Yo San University of Traditional Chinese Medicine, Los Angeles, USA

Li Wan-ling (李云宁)
Qi Gong and TCM Translator, Beijing, China

Liang Li-na (梁丽娜)**, Ph.D. TCM**
Associate Professor of Ophthalmology, Eye Hospital of China Academy of Chinese Medical Sciences, Beijing, China

Liu Zhan-wen (刘占文)
Professor of Chinese Medicine, Beijing University of Chinese Medicine, Beijing, China

Lü Ming (吕明)
Professor of Tui Na, Changchun University of Chinese Medicine, Changchun, China

Mark L. Mondot, B.A. Chinese Language, L.Ac.
Translator and Editor, People's Medical Publishing House, Beijing, China

Jane Lyttleton, Hons, M Phil, Dip TCM, Cert Ac.
Lecturer, University of Western Sydney, Sydney, Australia

Julie Mulin Qiao-Wong (乔木林)
Professor of Chinese Medicine, Victoria University, Melbourne, Australia

Andy Rosenfarb, M.S. TOM, L.Ac.
Acupuncture Health Associates, New Jersey, USA

Paul F. Ryan, M.S. TCM, L.Ac.
Taihu Institute, Jiangsu, China

Martin Schweizer, Ph.D. Molecular Biology, L.Ac.
Emeritus Professor of Medicinal Chemistry, University of Utah, USA

Secondo Scarsella, MD, DDS
Visiting Professor of Tui Na, Nanjing University of TCM, China Department of Maxillofacial Surgery, San Salvatore Hospital, L'Aquila, Italy

Sun Guang-ren (孙广仁)
Professor of TCM Fundamentals, Shandong University of TCM, Jinan, China

Tsai Chun-hui, Ph.D.
Associate Professor of Pediatrics, School of Medicine, University of Colorado, Denver, USA

Tu Ya (图娅)
Professor of Acupuncture and Moxibustion, Beijing University of CM, Beijing, China

Wang Shou-chuan (汪受传)
Professor of TCM Pediatrics, Nanjing University of TCM, Nanjing, China

Wei Qi-ping (韦企平)
Professor of Ophthalmology, Beijing University of CM, Beijing

Preface

In the development of human civilization, countless efforts have been made to extend life. As early as the Qin Dynasty some 2000 years ago, Qin Shi Huang, the first emperor of feudal China, united the country and consolidated power, but failed to find the solution for immortality. Qin Shi Huang sent the alchemist Xu Fu across the sea to Japan, bringing with him 3000 virgin boys and girls. Thousands of years have passed, the virgin boys and girls have long gone, but no one has ever found the elixir for immortality. It remains only a pipe dream for generations that followed. In the *Book of the Late Han Dynasty (Hòu Hàn Shū, 后汉书)*, there is record of the famous doctor, Hua Tuo, who cured and saved many people during the chaotic time of the Three Kingdoms. Hua Tuo always said to his students that physical exercise would improve appetite and digestion. More importantly, it would promote the circulation of qi and blood and thus prevent disease, like the hinge of a door that would not rot if you turn it everyday. He also created a health exercise, *Wu Qin Xi* (The Five Animals Frolic), for people to practice everyday.

The ancients always said, "There are too few who live to the age of seventy (人活七十古来稀)." Modern civilization and technology provide us much more time and space to seek longevity and a higher quality of life. There is no doubt that a healthy body is a basic requirement to reach these goals. In pursuing physical health, people have used numerous ways and practices, such as qigong, wu shu, health exercises, and many other methods. Among all physical exercises, traditional Chinese tai ji quan is unique and is attracting more and more attention because of its many strengths, including its scientific principles, practicality and efficiency. Tai ji quan is moderate in intensity, integrates both dynamic and static training, can be practiced according to personal needs and conditions, and provides great health benefits.

Tai ji quan integrates the essence of traditional Chinese culture, philosophy, and wu shu. The principles of tai ji quan are based on the philosophy of tai ji, the theory of yin and yang, the principles of wu shu and qi gong, and the theory of channels and collaterals from traditional Chinese medicine. Using a more precise description, tai ji quan is a physical exercise, a form of wu shu guided by a combination of traditional Chinese philosophy, and the study of human physiology. It has an irreplaceable role in promoting health. At the same time, the term "tai ji" has a philosophical interpretation of opposing but unified matter in motion. Therefore, the term "tai ji quan" reflects the exquisite quality of its techniques and profoundness of its theory. It is also why tai ji quan is often referred to as "the marital art of philosophy." Those who intend to practice tai ji quan should not only understand the meaning of the term and the nature of the exercise, but also need to study its philosophy and theory. Furthermore, they need to learn and understand its patterns and skills through daily practice.

As a form of wu shu, the early development of tai ji quan was focused on physical training and practical combat. However, it is important to note that tai ji quan absorbed the theories and principles of ancient Chinese health cultivation. It requires a calm mind and relaxed body during practice, with an upright but comfortable body structure. Tai ji quan emphasizes guiding body movements by mental intention, and sinking the qi to the elixir field (*dān tián*) in the lower abdomen. It is a health exercise combining elements of motion and stillness, external and internal, softness and hardness, and upper and lower. It emphasizes the application of mind instead of force to lead qi to circulate smoothly throughout the body. This will free the channels and collaterals, promote blood circulation, improve the physique, and enhance resistance to disease. Tai ji quan developed into a number of different schools including Chen, Yang, Wú, Wǔ and Sun, providing a variety of techniques and routines. Factors such as a more hectic lifestyle, changing living and working environments, and the stress of competitive and interpersonal relationships are directly or indirectly impairing people's healths. This results in increased cancer rates, metabolic disorders, and chronic fatigue syndrome, among other illnesses. Tai ji quan can play an important role in resisting these diseases and eliminating pathogenic factors. In short, it can improve quality of life by promoting health and preventing and treating disease. For all these reasons and with its solid theoretical and technical foundation, tai ji quan has already become the most popular form of wu shu practiced in China, and is soon becoming everyone's favorite health-promoting exercise.

We believe that with increased demand for a better quality of life, traditional tai ji quan has proven to play a more significant role in promoting health and prolonging life, and will become even more popular and appreciated. In recent decades, the ancient practice of tai ji quan is gaining popularity around the world and has become a favorite among wu shu enthusiasts.

The Yang Style 40 Movements Routine is used for demonstration purposes in this book. Yang style is one of the major schools of Chinese tai ji quan. The Yang Style 40 Movements Routine is a competition routine compiled and approved by tai ji quan experts at the invitation of the China Wu Shu Research Institute. It has all the characteristics of the Yang style, being slow, soft and fluid, with movements that are extended, clear, nimble, steady, simple, and dignified. It is also well-structured, which enhances comprehensive training. Regarding competition, its movements, content, timing, and structure all fully comply with wu shu competition regulations. As for health cultivation, it enhances coordination, consistency, flexibility, and mind-body harmony. The movements are simple and clear with no vigorous actions. It is also easy to learn and practice, appreciated by tai ji quan fans, and is becoming very popular. We have taught tai ji quan in foreign countries since the early 1990's. Most of our students think that the 24 Movements Routine is too simple, while the 88 Movements Routine is too complicated for beginners. We demonstrate the 40 Movements Routine in this book since it is simple to learn, of moderate complexity, and is suitable for foreign students. It has sufficient depth to enable a beginner to acquire the basic skills and patterns of tai ji quan, yet allows a beginner to develop an understanding of more complicated theories in a step-by-step approach.

Hu Zhen & Xu Shi-zu
July 2010

Table of Contents

Chapter 1 Introduction   1

Section 1 Basic Concepts of Tai Ji Quan... 1
Section 2 Theory of Tai Ji Movement 2
    1. Tai Ji Holism.. 2
    2. Concept of Constant Motion 3
    3. Concept of Equilibrium.. 3

Chapter 2 History of Tai ji Quan and Establishment of Different Schools   5

Section 1 Origin of Tai Ji Quan 5
Section 2 Formation and Development of Tai Ji Quan 6
Section 3 Establishment and Development of Different Schools 8
Section 4 Popularization of Tai Ji Quan.. 9

Chapter 3 The Principles of Tai Ji Quan   11

Section 1 Natural Laws of Life: Tai Ji and Yin-Yang Theory 11
    1. Opposition of Yin and Yang.. 11
    2. Interdependence of Yin and Yang... 12
    3. Reciprocal Growth and Decline of Yin and Yang 13
    4. Inter-transformation of Yin and Yang 14
Section 2 Source of Life Energy: Tai Ji and Qi 14
Section 3 Master of Life Activities: Tai Ji and Essence-Spirit Theory 15

Chapter 4 Tai Ji Quan and Health   17

Section 1 Effect of Tai Ji Quan on Heart Function.. 17

Section 2 Effect of Tai Ji Quan on Spleen-Stomach Function 19

Section 3 Effect of Tai Ji Quan on Lung Function 20

Section 4 Effect of Tai Ji Quan on Kidney Function 21

Chapter 5 Characteristics of Different Styles and How to Choose a Style   23

Section 1 How to Choose a Style as a Beginner 23

Section 2 Characteristics of Chen Style Tai Ji Quan 24

Section 3 Characteristics of Yang Style Tai Ji Quan 25

Section 4 Characteristics of Wǔ Style Tai Ji Quan 26

Section 5 Characteristics of Wú Style Tai ji Quan 26

Section 6 Characteristics of Sun Style Tai Ji Quan 27

Chapter 6 Basic Postures and Requirements of Tai Ji Quan   28

Section 1 Basic Postures of Tai Ji Quan 28

   1. Basic Hand Formations 28

   2. Basic Body Postures 28

   3. Basic Footwork 29

Section 2 Basic Requirements for Tai Ji Quan Practice 34

   1. Requirements for Body Movements 34

      ☯ Correct Body Posture

      ☯ Relaxation, Peace and Naturalness

      ☯ Waist is the Key for All Movements

      ☯ Smooth, Flexible and Coherent

   2. Requirements for the Mind 36

      ☯ Correct Physical Structure

      ☯ Faintly Discernible

   3. Requirements for the Breath 36

      ☯ Natural Breathing

      ☯ Abdominal Breathing

Section 3 Common Problems and Solutions Found in Teaching Tai Ji Quan 37

   1. Inability to Relax: Causes and Solutions 37

2. Inability to Concentrate: Causes and Solutions 37

Chapter 7 Yang Style 40 Movements Tai Ji Quan Routine   **39**

Ready Posture 预备势 39

Movement 1: Opening 起势 39

Movement 2a: Step Forward & Ward Off 上步掤 40

Movement 2b: Grasp the Sparrow's Tail 揽雀尾 40

Movement 3: Single Whip 单鞭 42

Movement 4: Raise Hands & Step Forward 提手上势 43

Movement 5: White Crane Spreads Wings 白鹤亮翅 44

Movement 6: Twist Step & Brush Knee 搂膝拗步 45

Movement 7: Hands Strum the Lute 手挥琵琶 48

Movement 8: Parry & Punch 搬拦捶 48

Movement 9: Apparent Close 如封四闭 49

Movement 10: Diagonal Flying 斜飞势 50

Movement 11: Fist Under the Elbow 肘底捶 51

Movement 12: Step Back & Whirl Arms 倒卷肱 53

Movement 13: Work Shuttle (Left & Right) 左右穿梭 55

Movement 14: Part the Wild Horse's Mane (Left & Right) 左右野马分鬃 56

Movement 15: Wave Hands Like Clouds 云手 58

Movement 16: Single Whip 单鞭 59

Movement 17: Pat High on Horse 高探马 60

Movement 18: Right Heel Kick 右蹬脚 60

Movement 19: Double-strike the Ears 双风贯耳 61

Movement 20: Left Toe Kick 左分脚 62

Movement 21: Turn Body & Heel Kick 转身蹬脚 63

Movement 22: Needle at Sea Bottom 海底针 64

Movement 23: Deflect through the Back 闪通背 65

Movement 24: White Snake Spits Tongue 白蛇吐信 65

Movement 25: Right Slap Kick 右拍脚 66

Movement 26: Subdue Tiger (Left & Right) 左右伏虎势 67

Movement 27: Crouch Down (Right) 右下势 69

Movement 28: Golden Cock Stands on One Leg 金鸡独立 70

Movement 29: Bow Stance & Strike Groin 弓步指裆 71

Movement 30: Grasp the Sparrow's Tail 揽雀尾 72

Movement 31: Single Whip 单鞭 72

Movement 32: Crouch Down (Left) 左下势 72

Movement 33: Step Forward to Seven Stars 上步七星 73

Movement 34: Step Back & Straddle the Tiger 退步跨虎 73

Movement 35: Turn Body & Lotus Kick 转身摆莲 74

Movement 36: Bend Bow to Shoot Tiger 弯弓射虎 75

Movement 37: Parry & Punch 搬拦捶 76

Movement 38: Apparent Close 如封四闭 77

Movement 39: Cross Hands 十字手 77

Movement 40: Closing 收势 78

Chapter 8 Common Mistakes in Tai Ji Quan Practice   79

1. Feet Not Parallel 79

2. Knees Overly Bent 79

3. Waist Bent 80

4. Shoulders Shrugged and Elbows Raised 81

5. Head is Dropped or Raised 82

6. Underarms are Constricted 82

7. Body is Unsteady when Shifting Weight 82

8. Body Leans while Shifting Weight 82

Appendix Yang Style Tai Ji Quan Routines   83

1. The 8 Movements Routine 八式太极拳拳谱 83

2. The 16 Movements Routine 十六式太极拳拳谱 83

3. The 24 Movements Routine 二十四式太极拳拳谱 83

4. The 32 Movements Routine 三十二式太极拳拳谱 84

5. The 48 Movements Routine 四十八式太极拳拳谱 85

6. The 88 Movements Routine 杨式88式太极拳拳谱 86

7. The Yang Style Old Frame Dynamic 128 Movements Routine
杨式老架动功太极拳128式拳谱 88

References　　　　　　　　　　　　　　　　　　　　　　**92**

Index　　　　　　　　　　　　　　　　　　　　　　**93**

1

Chapter 1 Introduction

Section 1 Basic Concepts of Tai Ji Quan

Tai ji quan is a shining treasure rooted in the soil of traditional Chinese culture. Being an indispensable part of traditional Chinese wu shu, tai ji quan is a product of how ancient Chinese used traditional philosophy to guide the martial arts. With its unique form of expression, tai ji quan has added rich meaning to traditional Chinese culture. It is the reflection of accumulated wisdom of not only the Chinese, but also of the entire human race. Tai ji quan is based on the principle of tai ji, which is ubiquitous in nature, combining the opposing but unified tai ji movements of yin and yang, and the traditional Chinese medical theories of *zang-fu* (viscera and bowels), and channels and collaterals, while finding expression in wu shu form via body movement.

For beginners, understanding the meaning of the term "tai ji quan" is a prerequisite for getting a clear direction for how to learn tai ji quan. The practice of tai ji quan must follow certain fundamental theories and principles.

The name "tai ji quan" comes from terminology used in traditional Chinese philosophy and theories about "tai ji." The term "tai ji" was first seen in *Commentary on the Classic of Changes-The Essay Series* (*Yì Zhuàn-Xì Cí*,易传-系辞), and reflects the height of learning with respect to ancient Chinese philosophy, especially that of the *Classic of Changes* (*Yì Jīng*, 易经). In Chinese, the word "*tài* (太)" means reaching and the word "*jí* (极)" means extreme. Therefore, tai ji means "reaching the extreme" and "not opposing each other." Another tai ji concept includes the idea of a boundless extreme in space and time. It can also mean reaching the highest realm. Tai ji can be larger than infinity and smaller than infinitesimal. With further observation and understanding of nature and the universe, tai ji has gradually been used to interpret the patterns of change in the universe and the endless cycles of life.

Fig.1 Tai Ji Diagram:

Black is yin; white is yang

The profundity of tai ji is how tai ji movement gives birth to two opposing but unified aspects of a whole: yin and yang (Fig. 1). This concept is the soul of tai ji theory. Tai ji quan is an artistic sport that consciously guides body movement in accordance with fundamental laws governing matter in motion. It is an advanced and sophisticated exercise harmonizing the body's interior and exterior, and generating force from inside to outside. Famous tai ji quan master Zheng Man-qing (郑曼青) described it as "swimming on land". It is not simply a set of combat techniques, but an artistically rich study with its own unique style. Again, practitioners must understand and study the meaning, nature, philosophies, and theories of tai ji quan. Only then can they put learning and understanding into practice, experience its unique character, and master its beautiful movements that are like flowing water and floating clouds. In another words, tai ji quan is an activity based on the opposing but unified changes of yin and yang generated through tai ji movement. In sum, it involves exercising the body internally and externally, which leads to two different manifestations: an internal and an external dynamic structure. True tai ji quan is practiced from interior to exterior, with internal dominating external body movements. In other words, tai ji movements start internally to lead the body's movements to achieve interior and exterior coordination and unification. The practitioner must synchronize and harmonize internal and external movements in tai ji quan practice. An exterior structure that is not coordinated with internal tai ji movement is not the true tai ji quan and thus will not achieve the desired results of tai ji quan practice.

Section 2 Theory of Tai Ji Movement

Tai ji quan is a study of human body movement in accordance with the principle of tai ji movement, which manifests as the transformation of yin and yang. To learn tai ji quan, we should understand the theory of tai ji movement first, including: tai ji holism, the concept of constant motion, and the concept of equilibrium. These theories and concepts have been applied throughout the history of tai ji quan practice and have been verified by practitioners since its creation. To master tai ji quan, one must have a comprehensive understanding of these superb theories and concepts; only in so doing can a practitioner explore tai ji quan's profound wisdom.

1. Tai Ji Holism

In their long observation and exploration of life and natural mysticism, the ancients gradually developed concepts about holism. Such holistic concepts were connected with their understanding about the world's origin, emphasizing unity of man and nature. These ancient thoughts about tai ji holism provide a lively philosophical interpretation.

Concepts about holism can be interpreted in two ways. First, as a part of nature, humans should maintain a coordinated and harmonious relationship with their external environment. To explain more specifically, living in the external universe, nature provides us with bright sunshine, fresh air and clean water, all of which are essential for human survival. Any changes in nature will directly or indirectly influence the daily lives and physiological conditions of humans. For example, seasonal changes lead to climatic characteristics, such as the warmth of spring, heat of summer, coolness of autumn, and cold of winter, which directly affect the daily lives and activities of humans. Therefore, humans and nature are an interrelated and inseparable unified whole. During tai ji quan practice, one way practitioners can harmonize themselves with the universe is by regulating their breathing.

The second concept about holism concerns the human body. It is seen as an organic whole, with all the component parts of the body interrelated and interdependent; they cannot be divided into independent structures. Every part of the body, even as small as a single tissue, is interrelated and cannot be isolated; a single change will affect all the other parts. Such thought applies to all tai ji theories and is critical in guiding tai ji quan practice. For example, tai ji quan tightly integrates the vertex of the head, hips, heart (mind), eyes, ears, hands, feet, and waist, forming a unified whole which changes and moves together flexibly. When one part moves, all parts move; when one part is still, all parts become still.

In tai ji quan practice, force (*jìn*, 劲) originates from the heels, with the waist as the key to all movements. Force goes upward to the legs, then to the back of the trunk and then the shoulders, and finally to the fingertips. The process of force going upward from feet to waist to fingers is thoroughly connected and well integrated with the internal organs, sinews and bones, skin, muscles, channels and collaterals, and every part of the body. Holism is fully reflected in tai ji quan, in which every posture and movement combines emptiness and solidity, upper and lower, forward and backward, and internal and external dynamics of the body.

2. Concept of Constant Motion

From observations of nature, we have learned about the movement of celestial bodies, seasonal changes, the tides of rivers, lakes and oceans, and the activities of birds and animals. These endless changes have allowed mankind to gradually understand that everything in the universe is in continuous and endless motion and transformation. Through long-term observation of natural phenomena, mankind has learned that the movement and transformation of matter is continuous. Movement is seen as a basic form of material existence, and an eternally present cosmic phenomenon.

The concept of constant motion indicates that everything in the dynamic world is in perpetual and endless motion and change. It is believed that everything in the universe, including the entire natural world and the human body, undergoes endless movement, change and qi transformation. The Earth is surrounded by a gaseous atmosphere and revolves in a continuous and specific pattern. The Earth revolves around the Sun from in a westward direction, and it rotates on its own axis eastwardly. These movements continue endlessly and appear in the changes of season as well as changes in all living things.

The concept of constant motion is one of tai ji quan's most important. The ancients observed the movement of celestial bodies and characterized tai ji movements into four basic patterns: ascending, descending, exiting and entering. These movements are endless and similar to how qi flows among celestial bodies. The movement mechanism of ascending, descending, exiting and entering is a universal phenomenon for matter and can only manifest on a material basis. However, the phenomenon is different among different types of matter because of differences in space and time.

As a part of nature, man is like everything else in the universe and is in a state of perpetual motion and change. Qi movement inside the body is everywhere and ever present. Because of its continuous circulation and changes within channels and collaterals, qi can function normally to nourish the organs internally, and the skin and muscles externally. Therefore, qi movement is eternal for both animate and inanimate matter. It is this eternal movement that leads to various and endless changes. Continuous movement is the motivating force for the origin and development of everything in the universe. If matter is still, without any motion, no generation and change can occur, and life would extinguish. Tai ji quan requires practitioners to move in a continuous and smooth way without any breaks in order for power to reach all areas of the body, including the limbs.

3. Concept of Equilibrium

Everything and every phenomenon in nature shows two opposing aspects. The normal state of the two opposing aspects is to maintain a dynamic balanced relationship. Opposing aspects, such as up and down, left and right, heaven and earth, dynamic and static, exit and entry, ascending and descending, day and night, cold and hot, all depend on each other for existence, showing an interdependent relationship. This is what is implied in the concept of equilibrium.

The practice of tai ji quan is also a constantly changing process of dynamic equilibrium. During practice, different parts of the body, including the internal and external, front and back, exterior and interior, upper and lower, and empty and solid steps, should all maintain a dynamic equilibrium in order to achieve optimal results. The practitioner needs to learn how to activate the entire body with a single tiny movement, and to become motionless when any part of the body is still. Every part of the body continually shifts between empty and solid movements, while the entire body maintains a dynamic equilibrium. To achieve such a skill level as soon as possible, tai ji quan elders left us with many techniques. For example, the body is described as a cross. To harmonize interior and exterior, the four ends of the horizontal and vertical lines forming the cross should be in balance. The horizontal line of the cross, forming the two shoulders, should be kept level horizontally to prevent the body from leaning sideways in practice. The vertical line of the cross, representing the line linking DU 20 (*bǎi huì*, 百会; located on the vertex) and the bottom of the torso (tailbone), should be kept vertical during practice in order to fulfill the requirement of "pushing the vertex upward" and "relaxing the tail." The intersection of the cross is in front of the thoracic vertebrae, which is the center of the body and key to tai ji quan practice. Only with correct body posture can the external body structure integrate with internal power to achieve interior-exterior harmony. When structure and posture are correct, central equilibrium is attained and tai ji quan's unique characteristics are realized. However, to attain internal power and correct posture is a difficult process full of hardship. The aforementioned results can only be accomplished through persistent study and diligent practice. To meet the requirements of tai ji quan, every single movement should be performed flawlessly, achieving a feeling of roundness and fullness. In other words, one must achieve opposing yet unified equilibrium with movements that appear circular. These characteristics also help explain the meaning of the term "tai ji" and why the practice is called "tai ji quan".

Chapter 2
History of Tai Ji Quan and Establishment of Different Schools

As a country with a five-thousand-year history, Chinese culture embodies a deep understanding of human health. From ancient times until now, the Chinese have created a splendid history that has been well documented. From ancient documents we find that in all aspects of traditional Chinese culture, whether Daoism, Buddhism, Confucianism, medicine, etc., there are a wealth of studies and practices about promoting health and strengthening the body. Wu shu has always been an important way for the Chinese to accomplish this. Tai ji quan is unique and special among all wu shu practices. According to various studies, the history of tai ji quan development can be divided into four phases.

Section 1 Origin of Tai Ji Quan

The emergence of tai ji quan on Chinese soil was not by chance. Hua Tuo, a famous doctor in the Three Kingdoms period, created *Wŭ Qín Xì* (Five Animal Frolic), providing people a way to promote health and strengthen the body in harmony with the laws of the nature. Xu Xuan-ping in the Tang Dynasty was a woodsman, but he fasted and rarely ate anything, "walked as fast as running horses", and wrote excellent poetry. Li Bai saw one of his works, thought it was a "divine poem", went to Xu's home several times, but never found him. In many folk tales, Xu was skilled in wu shu and played an important role in the origin of tai ji quan. However, there are not many records about his life, and he did not leave anything in writing.

There are many historical records about the famous master Zhang San-feng (张三丰). The well-known writer of wu shu tales, Mr. Jin Yong[1], has described Zhang San-feng as the founder of tai ji quan, a story very popular among modern Chinese. Zhang's original name was Zhang Tong. He was also known as Zhang Jun-shi or Zhang Jun-bao, and was a Han[2] Chinese Daoist born in Yi Zhou, Liao Dong (today's Fu Xin in Liaoning Province). According to studies on Daoism, Zhang San-feng lived around A.D. 1314-1320 to 1417 (Yan You years of the Yuan Dynasty to the Yong Le 15th year of the Ming Dynasty). Zhang was a magistrate when he was young, and saw three peaks while touring Baoji Mountain. The mountain was beautiful and Zhang really liked it, so he named himself San-feng since in Chinese the word "*fēng* (丰)" sounds like the word peak (*fēng*, 峰) and "*sān* (三)" means three. Zhang San-feng founded a new school of Daoism on Wudang Mountain (武当山) —the San Feng School, greatly influencing the development of Daoism. As the founder of Wudang wu shu, Zhang had excellent martial arts skills. He is known as the father of *nèi jiā quán* (internal wu shu). There are two stories about how Zhang San-feng created internal wu shu:

The first theory is that it is taught by the Zhen Wu God. According to records in *Epitaph of Wang*

---

[1] Jin Yong: The pen name of Louis Cha, co-founder of Ming Pao (one of the most popular newspaper in Hong Kong) and a famous modern Chinese novelist.

[2] Han: The main ethnic group in China.

Zheng-nan (*Wáng Zhēng Nán Mù Zhì Míng*, 王征南墓志铭) and *Records of Ning Bo Governmental Office* (*Níng Bō Fǔ Zhì*, 宁波府志), one night on a trip to Bian Jing (the capital city at that time), Zhang San-feng had a dream about the Zhen Wu God teaching him martial arts. At dawn of the second morning he was attacked by a group of robbers, and defeated them using the martial arts taught by the Zhen Wu God. Since then, Zhang San-feng has been known for his outstanding martial arts skills.

The second possible origin of internal wu shu is that is the result of inspiration drawn from the fight between a bird and a snake. The tale of Zhang San-feng's witness of the fight has been passed down through the generations. In this story, Zhang San-feng saw a bird fighting with a snake on La Ta Cliff. Whenever the bird flew up and down to try to attack the snake, the snake twisted and wiggled to dodge it. After quite a while, the bird grew exhausted and flew away, the snake was free and slid away into the grass. Zhang San-feng was inspired by the scene, believing that softness can overcome hardness and stillness can restrain movement; he created the internal martial arts by imitating the movements of the snake.

The names of the techniques and movements and the arrangement of routines are all based on Daoist classics. Internal martial arts are a profound study with many different schools, but they all regard Zhang San-feng as their founding father. Also, different schools share the same characteristics, emphasizing internal practice, the coordination and harmony of intention (*yì*, 意), qi (气) and force (*lì*, 力) according to the principles of yin and yang. The postures should be stable and the movements done with a vigorous strength, in a calm and effortless manner. When applied in combat, the principle is to overcome hardness with softness, and restrain movement with stillness.

The internal martial arts created by Zhang San-feng can "cultivate health internally and resist evil externally". These practices can enhance willpower, cultivate the mind, strengthen the body, promote health, and be used for self-defense. Therefore, the internal martial arts created by Zhang San-feng is a precious cultural legacy left for humanity, and one that will always be appreciated by succeeding generations.

Before the Qing Dynasty, tai ji quan was only a part of internal martial arts and not an independent form of practice. Since the Qing Dynasty, it has gradually developed into an independent practice and study.

Although there are many arguments about the origin of tai ji quan, we can say it is a product of Chinese culture, an accumulation of human wisdom, and a major gift to mankind for promoting health.

Section 2 Formation and Development of Tai Ji Quan

The development of tai ji quan dates mainly from the end of the Ming Dynasty to the beginning of the Qing Dynasty, and from the time of Chen Wang-ting to Cheng Chang-xing. During this period, the heritage of tai ji quan was passed down for five generations and evolved into Chen style tai ji quan. According to a study by Mr. Tang Hao, an historian of wu shu history, tai ji quan was first practiced in the Chen family at Chenjiagou (Chen Village) in Wen County, Henan Province.

According to records in *The Genealogy of the Chen Family* (*Chén Shì Jiā Pǔ*, 陈氏家谱), Chen Wang-ting was the founder of Chen style tai ji quan. Chen Wang-ting, born into a family of wu shu practitioners, was the ninth generation in his family to practice wu shu. Chen's father, Chen Fu-min, and grandfather, Chen Si-gui, were both fond of wu shu. Chen Wang-ting began to practice wu shu from

Fig.2 The Development of Tai Ji Quan and Interrelationship Between Different Schools

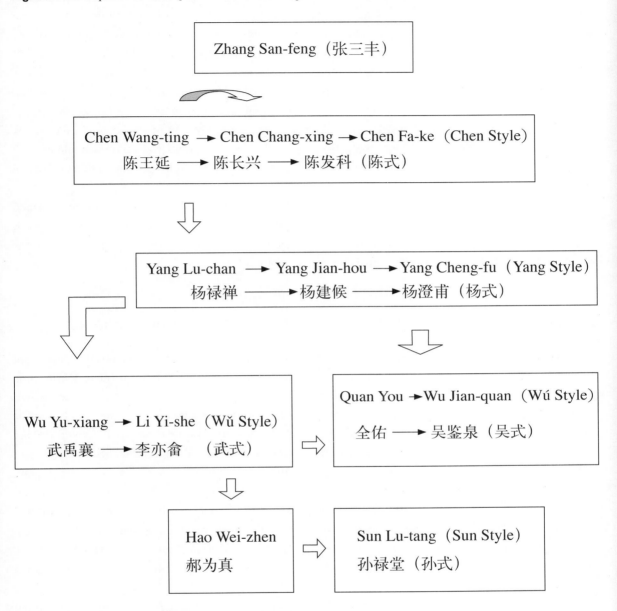

early childhood. The Ming Dynasty was overthrown when Chen Wang-ting was in the prime of life, when he excelled at wu shu. Chen Wang-ting had severe asthma in his old age, but could still do farm work and continued practicing wu shu. From available information, the creation of tai ji quan occurred around the 17th Century, about 30 years after the end of the Ming Dynasty in 1644 A.D.

After a long time of practice, study, and exploration, Chen Wang-ting created and developed tai ji quan on the foundation of the wu shu practice passed on within the family. Since Chen first created tai ji quan, all of his family descendants have practiced the art, no matter young or old, male or female, greatly influencing the Chen's of Chenjiagou.

During the past three centuries, the population in Chenjiagou increased considerably, with more and more people there practicing tai ji quan; their skills and techniques have become better and better, and many masters have emerged. The routines of tai ji quan have been changed with continuous innovations. There were mainly seven different routines from Chen Wang-ting's time until the fifth generation (after the time of Chen Chang-xing). There was the original 108 *cháng quán* routine (long fist routine) and the second to fifth tai ji quan routines; these were gradually abandoned and are rarely practiced anymore. The first and second tai ji quan routines have become the most popular. There are old frame and new frame versions for the Chen style first routine that have larger and less difficult movements compared to the original ones. During this period the Zhao Bao style emerged, with Chen Qing-ping as the representative for this style. It played an important role in the popularization of tai ji quan. The complex routines of Chen Wang-ting have been gradually simplified in order to popularize tai ji quan and make it more suitable for more people, an indication that tai ji quan has moved toward popularization and health promotion.

The initial development of Chen style tai ji quan was completed during this period and formed the prototype of modern tai ji quan. There are many opinions on the origin of tai ji quan. However, after Chen Chang-xing, its development and how it was named is clear and generally accepted. All the various schools of tai ji quan were established on this common foundation.

Section 3 Establishment and Development of Different Schools

The establishment and development of different schools was a long process, from the time Yang Lu-chan started learning wu shu to Sun Lu-tang's establishment of Sun style tai ji quan. During this period, the Yang, Wú, Sun and Wǔ styles were created and developed, while the Chen style completed its consolidation. The five main schools developed into what we now practice.

Yang Lu-chan (1799-1872) was a student of Chen Chang-xing, and learned Chen style tai ji quan from him. Based on the Chen Style Old Frame 1st Routine, Yang gradually developed his own style and characteristics after many years of hard practice and study. After going to Beijing to teach tai ji quan, Yang Lu-chan modified the original tai ji quan routines to make it more suitable for the public and founded Yang style tai ji quan. During this process, his third son, Yang Jian-hou (1839-1917), modified it and created the Middle Frame Routine. Yang Jian-hou's third son, Yang Cheng-fu (1883-1936), eventually developed the Large Frame Routine. The Large Frame's movements are extended, simple and elegant in style, with no vigorous movements. It has been the most popular among all Yang style routines.

A master emerged from the students of the Yang family during this period named Wu Jian-quan (1870-1942). He was from Da Xing County in Hebei Province and created Wú style tai ji quan. Wu's father, Quan You (1834-1902), was a Manchu[3]. Wu Jian-quan adopted the Han culture and changed his last name to Wu. He learned the Large Frame Routine from Yang Lu-chan and the Small Frame from his son, Yang Ban-hou (1837-1892), and was famous for his soft power. When Wu Jian-quan taught at the Beijing Sports Research Institute (北京体育研究社), he removed the jumping, repetitions, power emission (*fā jìn*)[4] and more vigorous movements from the small frame tai ji quan routine. He emphasized slow, soft, fluid and smooth movements with characteristics similar to the Yang style. Wú style routines are performed at

---

[3] Manchu: one of the ethnic groups in China.
[4] *Fā jìn* (发劲) describes a sudden emission or release of power while doing a technique such as a punch or kick.

an even and consistent pace. The movements are small, compact, calm and comfortable, with no vigorous moves or jumps. The Wú style developed into southern and northern schools. The southern school followed Wu Jian-quan's lineage; the main successors were Wu Gong-zao, Wu Gong-yi, Wu Ying-hua, Ma Yue-liang, and others. The northern school followed Wang Mao-zhai's lineage; the main successors were Zhao Tie-an, Yang Yu-ting, and others; a later generation included Zhao An-xiang, Li Jing-wu, Wang Pei-sheng, and others.

Wu Yu-xiang (1812-1880) learned Chen style old frame tai ji quan from Yang Lu-chan, and new frame from Chen Qing-ping. He not only practiced hard, but also earnestly studied the tai ji quan classics, practicing in strict accordance with *Treatise on Tai Ji Quan* (*Tài Jí Quán Lùn*, 太极拳论), and eventually created *Wǔ* style tai ji quan. The style was further modified by Li Yi-she (1832-1892), who developed it into a final version of the Wǔ style. The Wǔ style is similar to the Yang and Chen styles, but the movements and structure are unique. It has its own characteristics and complicated theories. Wǔ style techniques can be summed up in four words: initiation, continuity, opening, and closing, with emphasis on opening, closing, and substantial (solid) and insubstantial (empty) postures and actions. The structure of the postures is compact, innovative, and unique.

Sun Lu-tang (1861-1892) started to learn wu shu as a child and was very good at *xíng yì quán* (形意拳) and *bā guà quán* (八卦拳), both internal marital arts. He subsequently learned Wǔ style tai ji quan from Hao Wei-zhen. Sun combined the strengths of the three and created Sun style tai ji quan. Sun style has high postures and lively footwork. It has a distinctive flavor with an emphasis on quick advances and retreats and coordinated opening and closing movements.

Chen Fa-ke (1887-1957), the great grandson of Chen Chang-xing, went to Beijing to popularize tai ji quan in 1928. He taught Chen style tai ji quan extensively. His techniques displayed relaxation, flexibility, explosive power, shaking force, spiraling energy, and foot stomping force. Through his persistent efforts, Chen Fa-ke enhanced the role of the Chen style in the development of tai ji quan and restored the glory of the style.

Except for the distinctive routines of Chen style, all the other four schools have similar routines and movement names; even their routine arrangements and sequence of movements are similar. All of these schools either enlarged or reduced the range of movements according to their own requirements to create their own styles. For example, Sun Lu-tang was very good at *xíng yì quán* and *bā guà zhǎng* and thus combined their techniques in his Sun style tai ji quan. Yang Cheng-fu created a large frame style tai ji quan since he had a tall and large physique. The Wǔ style was greatly influenced by Neo-Confucianism in the Song and Ming dynasties, and emphasized the application of philosophy in shaping its structure as well as for self-cultivation.

Section 4 Popularization of Tai Ji Quan

The popularization of tai ji quan occurred mainly from 1950 forward. During this period, the structures of different styles were more or less finalized with no significant changes. Every style gained in popularity and was promoted during this period. Since then, tai ji quan has been practiced in cities and in rural areas throughout China.

Beginning in 1956, the State Sports Commission of China, to better promote and popularize tai ji quan, created simplified tai ji quan and simplified tai ji sword routines. Created in 1979 were the 24

Movements Simplified Tai Ji Quan Routine, the 32 Movements Tai Ji Sword Routine, the 48 Movements Tai Ji Quan Routine, and others. The popularization of these routines greatly contributed to public enthusiasm for tai ji quan. After 1989, the State Sports Commission invited experts to create a number of competition routines, such as the 40 Movements Tai Ji Quan Competition Routine, the 42 Movements Integrated Tai Ji Quan Routine, the Wǔ Style Tai Ji Quan Competition Routine, and others. The competition routines provide the evaluation criteria used in tai ji quan practice and competition. All of these events contributed to the further development of tai ji quan. In 1994, the State Sports Commission of China proposed the "National Fitness Program." Because of tai ji quan's significant role in promoting health, the introduction of the program enhanced the popularity of tai ji quan throughout China, and led to greater public enthusiasm for practicing wu shu. With increasing international exchange, tai ji quan has gradually become a global health exercise. On March 22, 2001, the First World Tai Ji Quan and Health Conference was held in Sanya City, Hainan, where around 2000 people from all over the world participated in the competition, signifying the flourishing growth of tai ji quan's global appeal.

During this period, there have been no significant changes in the movements and arrangement of routines for the different styles. The new routines created by the State Sports Commission are mostly modeled after the traditional ones. The arrangement and flavor of the 24-, 48- and 42-movement routines are basically the same as the traditional ones, with only minor differences. The newly created routines retain the essence of the traditional ones, but reflect their own unique style and characteristics. The competition routines are also very similar to their originals, with no significant stylistic differences of their own. This is especially evident for the Yang, Wú and Sun styles. These are very similar and were mainly influenced by the Yang style. These and other factors, such as how competitions are conducted, may explain the popularity of Yang style tai ji quan.

As more and more people practice tai ji quan, research and development about it have been promoted. In particular, studies have been done on tai ji quan's health benefits, noteworthy combat techniques, and cultural foundations. Moreover, the unique benefits of tai ji quan have been proven scientifically. Our mission now is to create effective simplified routines while preserving traditional styles and features, and to get more people to practice tai ji quan.

Chapter 3   The Principles of Tai Ji Quan

Section 1 Natural Laws of Life: Tai Ji and Yin-Yang Theory

In *Commentary of the Classic of Changes – The Essay Series* (易传-系辞), it is said that "*Yi* has tai ji, which gives birth to two poles (易有太极，是生两仪)." The "two poles" here means that tai ji has two manifestations: yin and yang. That is, tai ji divides into two, gives birth to two opposing, but also unified and interdependent, entities. At the same time the two, yin and yang, can combine into one to form tai ji. The continual changes of the dividing and combining of tai ji and yin and yang are embodied in the natural laws of life that govern all living things in the universe. The patterns of tai ji movement reflect patterns of change and transformation within the universe (i.e., the movement of tai ji is a model of movement within the universe). It is a scientific model of change, and serves as a lighthouse guiding our way ahead in the ocean of scientific exploration.

The tai ji diagram drawn according to the principles of tai ji encompasses universal law that governs everything in existence. It is an important diagram that the ancient Chinese used to study universal principles. The tai ji diagram shows how the two opposing entities, yin and yang, move and change. From an in-depth study of the tai ji diagram, we learn that the changes of dividing and combining result from tai ji movement, which gives birth to yin and yang. Yin and yang are a paired couple in traditional Chinese philosophy. In the beginning, the concept simply implied two sides; the side facing the sun is yang, and the back side facing away from the sun is yin. Facing toward the sun make us feel warm and bright, with a lot of vitality; facing with our back in the shade always gives us a feeling of cold and dark, with a lack of vitality. Subsequently, the concept of yin and yang was extended to cover such opposing yet complimentary aspects as cold and warm, bright and dark, up and down, external and internal, restlessness and tranquility, etc.

In the tai ji diagram, yin on the right is represented by the color black, and "yang within yin" is represented by the white spot in the black. Yang on the left is represented by the color white, and "yin within yang" is represented by the black spot in the white.

Yin and yang theory is used to explain all change and transformation within the process of tai ji movement, and includes those between internal and external, empty and full, up and down, etc. Yin and yang are neither independent nor static, but are in a state of constant dynamic change; they are opposing, interdependent, reciprocal, and inter-transforming. These principles of change are the critical component of yin-yang theory.

1. Opposition of Yin and Yang

We believe that the world, including everything in it, is composed of matter, and that it is a material entity. From the tai ji diagram, we learn that everything in nature consists of mutually opposing yet unified aspects of yin and yang. The opposing paired aspects of yin and yang are not independent, but are unified. The opposing but unified relationship of yin and yang is the root cause of the origination, growth, change, and decline of everything in nature. Yin and yang not only imply that two things oppose or are opposite each other, but also imply two opposing aspects of the same thing. Things and phenomena that are warm, ascending, dynamic, outgoing, and bright are classified as yang; in contrast, those that are cold, descending, static, introverted, and dull are classified as yin. For example, the warmth of spring and the heat of summer represent yang, and the coolness of autumn and the coldness of winter represent yin. Similarly for water and fire, water is cold and flows downward in nature and thus can be classified as yin; fire is hot and burns upward in nature and thus can be classified as yang.

A practitioner is required to express the opposing nature of yin and yang throughout tai ji quan practice. In tai ji quan movements, the dynamic motions of the body are yang, and the static ones are yin; a movement is classified as yang if it is dynamic in the beginning and then becomes static. It can be classified as yin if a movement is static in the beginning and then becomes dynamic. Forward movements are yang and backward movements are yin; exterior is yang and interior is yin; ascending is yang and descending is yin; solid steps are yang and empty steps are yin[5]. As for the movements of the hands, the leading hand is yang and the assisting hand is yin.

2. Interdependence of Yin and Yang

In observing things and phenomena in mutual opposition, ancient Chinese philosophers learned that everything and every phenomenon in nature oppose as well as depend on each other. They believed that the opposition and interdependence of yin and yang is the nature of everything, and is a fundamental pattern of the universe. The interdependence of yin and yang means that yang relies on the yin and yin relies on the yang; they depend on each other for birth, growth, and existence. In other words, neither yin nor yang can exist alone without the other. For example, exterior is yang and interior is yin, if the exterior does not exist, you cannot explain what interior is; day is yang and night is yin, if there is no day, you cannot understand the concept of night. As for the human body, mental activities are yang and the physical body is yin; if the physical body does not exist, the mind cannot function. All of these examples explain that the two are interdependent; they exist or perish together. If there is no yin, there would be no yang, and vice versa. If yang disappears, yin will disappear at the same time.

A requirement of tai ji quan practice is to express the interdependence of yin and yang; for instance, one should coordinate the upper and lower body, as well as the left and right, and the internal and external. During tai ji quan practice, the hardness of yang and the softness of yin coexist in the same body. Yang is excessive if the movement is too rigid, and yin is excessive if the movement is too soft. In beginners, especially those who lack experience with the physical aspects, their moves tend to be rigid and their bodies stiff. To overcome this, practitioners need to practice the exercises with soft force first. After a certain period of persistent practice, stiffness can be softened and the body will become more and more agile; strength will be developed from softness, then strength will lead to softness again, and softness will result in strength again.

To recap, the principles and goals of tai ji quan practice are "to achieve hardness within softness, to use hardness and softness to support each other, and to use softness to restrain hardness (以柔中有刚，刚柔相济，最终到达以柔克刚)".

---

[5] Solid and empty steps refer to weighting. For example, the foot bearing more weight is considered full or solid; the one bearing less weight is empty.

3. Reciprocal Growth and Decline of Yin and Yang

Opposing but interdependent yin and yang are in a constant state of growth and decline; while yang is growing, yin is definitely declining, which we call the process of "yin decline with yang growth". When yin grows, yang inevitably declines, which is called the process of "yang decline with yin growth". This is the inevitable result of all movement, development and change. Take the four seasons of the year as an example; the climate changes from winter to spring then summer, and the temperature gradually changes from cold to hot. These changes illustrate a process of "yin decline with yang growth". When the climate changes from summer to autumn then winter, and the temperature gradually changes from hot to cold, this is the process of "yang decline and yin growth". The four seasons change with the reciprocal growth and decline of yin and yang with resulting transformations of cold, heat, warm, and cool. The reciprocal growth and decline of yin and yang is normally in dynamic equilibrium. If growth or decline exceeds the norm, balance is lost, and excess or deficiency of either yin or yang will occur. This imbalance will cause disease. The key to tai ji quan practice, therefore, is to maintain proper balance of the growth and decline of yin and yang. The ancients believed that conditions of yang without yin or yin without yang are both wrong. Those who can maintain yin and yang equilibrium are the real masters of tai ji quan. A song written by Chen Xin[6] in *Elaboration on General Introduction* (*Zǒng Lùn Fā Míng*, 总论发明) said:

"Pure yin with no yang is weak,
pure yang with no yin is stiff,
one portion of yin with nine portions of yang is a stick,
two portions of yin with eight portions of yang is simple combat,
three portions of yin with seven portions of yang is still stiff,
four portions of yin with six portions of yang is close to good,
only five portions of yin with five portions of yang,
with no imbalance of either yin or yang, is truly good."

纯阴无阳是软手，
纯阳无阴是硬手，
一阴九阳根头棒，
二阴八阳是散手，
三阴七阳由觉硬，
四阴六阳类好手，
唯有五阴并五阳，
阴阳无偏称妙手。

The main idea implied in this song is that the hardness of yang and softness of yin should be in proportional balance. If there is merely the softness of yin with no hardness of yang, there will be weakness; in contrast, if there is only the hardness of yang with no softness of yin, there will be an

---

[6] Chen style tai ji quan master and author of *The Illustrated Canon of Chen Family Tai Ji Quan.*

inability to yield. A perfectly balanced state is one with no excess of yang hardness or yin softness. A person who attains mastery is one who can keep the two in balance and not favor either side.

4. Inter-transformation of Yin and Yang

When yin or yang develops into a certain state under certain conditions, one can transform into the other, i.e., yin can change to yang and yang to yin. If the growth and decline of yin and yang is a process of quantitative change, then the inter-transformation of yin and yang is the process of qualitative change.

In tai ji quan movements, the process of shifting from solid step to empty step is a process of transformation of yang to yin; and shifting from empty step to full or solid step is the process of transformation of yin to yang. Under the guidance of this same principle, the process of shifting from external to internal or from upper to lower are both processes of transformation from yang to yin, while the processes of shifting from internal to external and from lower to upper are the processes of yin transforming to yang.

Section 2 Source of Life Energy: Tai Ji and Qi

As early as 5000 years ago, ancient Chinese philosophers had a basic understanding of natural phenomena, believing that tai ji is a turbid sphere filled with the primeval matter of life which they labeled original qi (*yuán qì*, 元气). They believed that original qi forms the world's most basic primeval matter, that everything in the universe is the result of qi movement and transformation, and that all movement and change is driven by qi. The practice of tai ji quan is not simply an exercise of the physical body, but more importantly physical exercises should reflect the body's movement of original qi. Original qi is the primary driving force of life activities, circulating throughout the body (including all the tissues, body parts and organs) and through the channels and collaterals; it activates and drives all the body's physiological activities. Therefore, original qi is the fundamental material element that maintains and critically affects human life activities and physiological functions. The physiological effects of qi are related to tai ji quan in the following three ways:

Activation effect: The body's growth and development, circulation of blood, distribution and metabolism of body fluids, and physiological function of organs, channels and collaterals all rely on qi activation to function properly. With the activation of qi, practitioners can have a continuous supply of power and energy. When qi moves and, for example, ascends or descends, exits or enters, the body is then able to ascend and descend, advance and retreat accordingly.

Warming effect: We should first make clear that original qi is the source of body heat, maintaining a relatively constant temperature in our bodies through its warming effect. If the original qi is dysfunctional and not warming, a person will display cold symptoms such as cold limbs, fear of cold, and a desire for warmth. In tai ji quan practice, because of qi's warming effect, practitioners are able to experience a warm and comfortable feeling during practice.

Defensive effect: Qi plays a defensive role in the body. The body's immune system is a complex one, influenced by the resultant functions of internal organs, channels, and collaterals. In *The Yellow Emperor's Internal Classic* (*Huáng Dì Nèi Jīng*, 黄帝内经), it is believed that external pathogenic factors cannot attack the body when one has sufficient resistance to disease; if invaded by pathogenic substances, it is due to the decline of one's ability to resist disease. This disease resistance is synonymous with "healthy qi (*zhèng qì*)." Therefore, qi is critical to the immune system. The defensive effect of qi is reflected in its defense of the body's exterior (such as the skin) to prevent the invasion of external pathogenic factors. If the defensive mechanism of qi is weakened, disease resistance will decline, and one will be easily attacked by pathogenic factors and get sick. Tai ji quan practice can stimulate original qi and promote qi circulation within the body to strengthen the body, prevent disease, and increase longevity.

Section 3 Master of Life Activities: Tai Ji and Essence-Spirit Theory

The concept of essence-spirit[7] originated from the ancients' understanding of life phenomena. When a male and a female have intercourse, a new life is produced and with it essence-spirit. To maintain the body's normal physiology, all the organs need to function normally; this includes the generation and distribution of qi, blood and body fluid, and all mental and emotional activities. All of these functions rely on the regulation and control of essence-spirit. The broad definition of essence-spirit covers all the manifestations of life activities; it is the governor of all physiological and mental activities. The narrower definition of essence-spirit encompasses the mind, the consciousness, and all thought processes.

Practitioners of tai ji quan should adjust their state of mind before practicing, be calm and peaceful, and eliminate all distracting thoughts in order to be ready for practice. Lead the movement of qi within the body with your conscious intention; in other words, all movements of the body should be of one mind (one heart). The mind should concentrated on regulating the original qi and leading it with conscious intention. Whether moving or staying still, slowing down or speeding up, all movements should follow your heart.

It bears repeating that in tai ji quan practice, you need to use your mental focus to lead the qi with conscious intention. Again, the practitioner should relax the entire body and let it be natural. Control the mind and be calm and peaceful without distracting thoughts. Do not use stiff and intense effort. Try not to be overly forceful; even a slight bit of it will cause the loss of naturalness and harmony, and tai ji will no longer be tai ji. Only in such a way can the body relax and be natural; then, original qi will be able to circulate within the body smoothly, and the body will be steady with the movements smooth and agile.

We know that the eyes can best reflect a person's emotional state. In tai ji quan, the practitioner should focus the mind, let the eyes follow the movement of the dominant hand, and neither look around nor allow the eyes to become too dull. The practitioner should activate the circulation of original qi by conscious intention to drive the body's movements. Only when a practitioner has total concentration can the body move accurately and gracefully. Once the practitioner becomes distracted or has distracting thoughts, the body mechanics, hand techniques, and footwork will be unnatural and fail to follow the principles of tai ji quan; this will then lead to deviations. Take the movement of "Single Whip" as an example; the practitioner should move slowly, focus the eyes on the left hand and not look around; when finishing the movement, shift the focus of the eyes to the left fingertips.

Before becoming familiar with the movements and developing a complete understanding of the

---

[7] Essence-spirit: *jīng shén*, 精神 in Chinese generally refers to the concept of mind or vigor when the two characters are used together in modern Chinese, while the character *jīng* means essence and the character *shén* means spirit.

practice, tai ji quan beginners tend to be too forceful, rigid, clumsy, and uncoordinated. Therefore, the first step for beginners is to learn how to lead internal qi movement with body movements. Once they get more used to the movements, they can lead the qi with conscious intention to guide and drive the body's movements. They can then cultivate both the interior and exterior simultaneously and achieve harmony of body and qi, form, and function.

Chapter 4　Tai Ji Quan and Health

The connection between tai ji quan practice, and health and longevity has always been a topic of discussion. Centuries of practice have proven that tai ji quan is an athletic activity that significantly promotes health and prevents and treats disease. In the tai ji quan classics, there an ancient saying, "What is the final purpose? It is the promise of long life and eternal youth, and to be forever young (详推用意终何在？延年益寿不老春)." From this we can understand tai ji quan's connection to health and longevity.

From a traditional Chinese medicine perspective, health depends on the sufficiency of a person's original qi. The practice of tai ji quan can regulate and train the mind, and promote the body's qi mechanism when guided by tai ji's principle of conscious intention. This will free the channels and collaterals, balance yin and yang, and harmonize qi and blood. It will improve intelligence, cultivate health, eliminate disease, and prolong life.

At the same time, in traditional Chinese medicine, if original qi is sufficient, the internal organs will function vigorously and a person will be healthy in both mind and body. Tai ji quan practice can calm the mind, relax the body, cultivate true qi (*zhēn qì*), regulate and promote qi movement, enhance the qi transformation function of internal organs, and promote the circulation of qi and blood. It can also free obstructed and stagnated channels and collaterals, and nourish the entire body. Therefore, it has the effect of increasing essence, blood, qi and vigor, and promoting both mental and physical wellbeing.

Section 1　Effect of Tai Ji Quan on Heart Function

In traditional Chinese medicine, the heart governs the blood and blood vessels. Normal blood circulation within the blood vessels greatly depends on normal heart function. Abnormal blood circulation or heart blood deficiency can both affect heart function. Another function of the heart is to govern the mind, consciousness and thinking. In tai ji quan practice, qi movement is guided by consciousness; qi movement activates body movement; and qi circulation follows conscious intention and activates blood circulation. As a result, according to tai ji quan treatises, "stagnation will be lessened when qi is distributed throughout the body (气遍周身不少滞)." Modern studies indicate that tai ji quan's orderly movements of opening and closing, and extending and contracting lead to the rhythmic contraction and relaxation of all muscles. This has the effect of spontaneously expanding capillaries, promoting venous return, reducing stress on the heart, and accelerating blood circulation. All this helps protect and promote heart function.

Cardio-cerebral vascular disease has become the "number one killer" in countries such as Europe, America and China. Better treatment and prevention are important missions for all. For the general public, to prevent cardio-cerebral vascular disease, besides quitting smoking and adjusting our daily diet, the most important method is regular physical exercise. Tai ji quan is one of the most effective for preventing cardio-cerebral vascular disease. The slow, soft, smooth and fluid movements of tai ji quan can increase blood vessel elasticity as well as neurovascular stability. The body can, therefore, better endure harmful external stimulation. Medical and scientific studies have confirmed that sports can increase good cholesterol (high-density lipoprotein) and help eliminate low-density lipoprotein, and thus reduce the risk of arteriosclerosis (hardening of arteries) and cardiovascular or cerebrovascular infarctions. In sum, tai ji quan is an ideal way to prevent cardio-cerebral vascular disease.

Another issue of concern is hypertension (high blood pressure). Except for secondary hypertension caused by other diseases, most hypertensive patients have primary hypertension. Besides taking medications, practicing tai ji quan is an effective way to prevent the spasm of small arteries since it can relax the mind and restore the function of the central nervous system. The elderly who regularly practice tai ji quan have a much lower average blood pressure and arteriosclerosis rate than the general population of elderly people.

Moreover, tai ji quan has wide-ranging regulatory effects on balancing the body's yin and yang. This results in a two-way regulatory effect to balance a person's condition. For example, tai ji quan practice can help both high and low blood pressure patients to return to normal blood pressure levels.

In traditional Chinese medicine, governing the spirit (mind) is another heart function; i.e., the heart regulates the mind, consciousness, and thought. Tai ji quan practice can restrain the mind and qi by training consciousness. It can coordinate internal organ functions by regulating the heart-*shen* (heart-spirit), and maintain and optimize their normal function in order to keep the body healthy. As is said in *The Yellow Emperor's Internal Classic*, "The subordinates are settled when the lord is bright; long life can be achieved if health is cultivated accordingly (主明则下安，以此养生则寿)." Tai ji quan can promote not only physical health, but also mental health. In the long-term observation of its societal impact, it has been found that tai ji quan has a very good effect in helping cultivate socially positive traits. For example, those who have practiced tai ji quan for a long time always show a gentle and even temperament, with a steady and calm demeanor. Therefore, tai ji quan is an excellent combination of cultural activity and physical exercise for promoting health and strengthening the body.

The effect of tai ji quan on mental health is mainly about the following:

Cultivate the mind: Tai ji quan emphasizes that both the body and mind should be relaxed, natural and tranquil during practice. Allow movements, guided by intention, to unfold. Internal qi movements should be in sync with external body movements to achieve a comfortable, carefree, and harmonious state of body and mind. This will help cultivate a sense of overall wellbeing. Practicing tai ji quan with proper background music will further relax the body and mind, help resolve mental fatigue, and help the practitioner develop a cheerful, optimistic, and positive character. When we were teaching at Burapha University in Thailand, there was a group of retired elderly students who consistently practiced tai ji quan daily. Everyday they looked refreshed and revitalized. Feeling good about themselves, they were happy, full of energy, and optimistic. Unlike many seniors, they were neither negative, sad, nor pessimistic.

Optimize personality: Tai ji quan practice requires unity of body and mind, and a steady and upright body posture. The movements should be slow and even, fluid and consistent, like that of floating clouds or flowing water. In motion, seek stillness; when still, find movement. Move in a way that integrates strength and softness, and emptiness and solidity. Regular tai ji quan practice will help those who are irritable, stingy, and suspicious to become steady, open-minded, calm, and optimistic. Also, persistent practice over a long time will help develop a spirit of perseverance, persistence and calmness to overcome problems such as laziness, indiscipline, and difficulty concentrating. This will develop positive personality and behavioral patterns. Therefore, tai ji quan is much more than just a martial art; embodied within is a far-reaching and profound mind-body philosophy. With continued tai ji quan practice, gradually the mind will become cultivated, and the personality optimized.

Prevent disease: Tai ji quan is an effective therapy for dealing with negative emotions such as anxiety, sadness, and emotional pain, and is effective in preventing psychosomatic illness caused by a variety of factors. This is because complete relaxation of mind-body tension is realized during practice, allowing the cerebral cortex sufficient rest and enhancing its function. It also increases body agility, sharpens reflexes, and reduces nervous system tension, thus preventing psychological diseases induced by mental stress. Therefore, tai ji quan is an effective method to promote mental health and help us acquire true wellbeing from the inside out.

Section 2 Effect of Tai Ji Quan on Spleen-Stomach Function

In traditional Chinese medicine, the spleen governs transformation and transportation within our body, and the stomach governs reception of food. "The spleen governs transformation and transportation" means that it has the function of digesting and absorbing food and drink, and distributing water and fluids throughout the body. "The stomach governs reception of food" means that the stomach has the function of receiving and digesting food, and then excreting the food residue through the intestines. The functioning of the spleen and stomach directly influences the qi dynamic of the body, and is especially critical for normal digestive function.

When performing tai ji quan, practitioners must maintain an upright body posture and a calm mind. Their upper and lower body movements should be coordinated, fluid and consistent, and synchronized with the movement of internal qi. In this way, body movement will lead the ascending, descending, exiting, and entering of qi. As a result, the whole body, including muscles of the chest, diaphragm, abdomen, back, waist, and channels and vessels will contract and relax in a rhythmic and orderly way. This not only exercises the entire body physically, but also has a self-massaging effect on the internal organs. It also promotes qi movement of the internal organs, optimizes the spleen's transformation and transportation function, the stomach's reception of food, and the liver's function in governing the free flow of qi. This has a positive influence on the digestive system, and is effective in preventing and treating related diseases. The spleen also provides nourishment for the muscles, which traditional Chinese medicine refers to as the function of the "spleen governs the flesh." Only when the spleen and stomach function properly in digesting and absorbing, can the muscles and bones acquire sufficient nourishment. This plus the smooth circulation of qi and blood driven by qi movement, and unobstructed flow within the channels and collaterals, will help relieve pain and treat muscle and joint disease.

When practicing tai ji quan, the waist should rotate over a wide range of motion to fully exercise the body's internal organs, including the liver, gallbladder, stomach and intestines. The movements should also be accompanied by proper breathing, which should be deep, long, fine and even. This will increase the diaphragm's range of up and down movements to massage the liver, gallbladder, stomach and intestines. These actions will then promote the circulation of qi and blood through the internal organs, and eliminate qi stagnation and blood stasis. These actions will improve the functioning of the aforementioned internal organs, especially gastrointestinal peristalsis and the secretion and regulation of digestive enzymes. These processes, therefore, play an important role in improving the function of the digestive system and preventing digestive diseases.

In addition, tai ji quan requires practitioners to touch the upper palate with the tip of the tongue during practice. This will increase the secretion of fluid (saliva), which is then swallowed and led downward to the elixir field (*dān tián*, 丹田). This technique greatly benefits digestion and enhances beauty. As the ancients indicated in their secrets of health cultivation: "Saliva is frequently generated at the tip of the tongue, and swallowed to the elixir field; it is delightful and fluid, and will preserve facial beauty after a hundred days of practice (津液频生在舌端，寻常咽津在丹田，于中畅美无凝滞，百日功灵可驻颜)." There is evidence to confirm that the application of deep abdominal breathing along with the continuous swallowing of fluid (saliva) can cultivate internal essence and qi. This will help people retain a youthful vitality and enhance appearance, add spring to their step, and relieve various aches and pains.

Section 3 Effect of Tai Ji Quan on Lung Function

In traditional Chinese medicine, the lung manages the body's qi. The lungs distributes and utilizes qi throughout the body by regulating breathing and the blood vessels. Oxygen is an essential substance for maintaining life activities. In daily life, humans rely on breathing to acquire oxygen for survival. Oxygen is inhaled into the lungs through the nose for gaseous exchange, then the carbon dioxide produced is exhaled. Oxygen is part of the physiological process of biologic oxidation, providing nutrients and energy to the body. On the one hand, the lungs transport oxygen all over the body via blood. Oxygen enables body tissues and cells to undergo the oxidative decomposition of proteins, fats, glucose, and other substances to produce nutrients the body needs for doing physical chores and daily activities. On the other hand, this metabolic process generates carbon dioxide that is harmful if left to accumulate in the body. Carbon dioxide is transported to the lungs via blood, and eliminated from the body by the lungs. This continuous respiration process ensures the supply of oxygen for energy transformation, sustains essential metabolism for life maintenance, and provides essential nutrients and energy for growth and development.

An internal requirement for tai ji quan practice calls for cultivating and activating the body's healthy qi (*zhèng qì*), regulating qi circulation within the channels and collaterals, and optimizing the gaseous exchange function of the lungs. This allows the body to optimize the usage of nutrients and energy. It requires practitioners to "sink qi to the elixir field", using even, fine, deep, and long abdominal breaths. By strictly following instructions as outlined, this method of breathing will enhance the movement of respiratory muscles, enlarge the thoracic cavity, maintain elasticity of the lungs, and thus increase vital capacity and improve respiratory function of the lungs. Hence, it is important to "relax the abdomen and activate the qi" during the entire practice. This will increase the capacity for gaseous exchange (pulmonary ventilation), and help optimize the lungs' physiological function.

In the course of daily living and work, one's health can be damaged by intense study, stressful work, and a fast-paced lifestyle—all of which can increase the body's oxygen consumption and result in oxygen deficiency in cells and tissues. Those with mild conditions may exhibit such symptoms as dizziness, palpitations, fatigue, shortness of breath, sluggishness, unclear thinking, and difficulty concentrating. Those with more severe symptoms may have dizziness with headache, nausea and vomiting, decreased blood pressure, clouded consciousness, or even unconsciousness. Those who are even worse off may suffer from shock or even die. Long-term deficiency of oxygen will cause fatigue, limb weakness, confusion, and irritability, and cause varying degrees of damage to body tissues and organs.

To recap, while practicing tai ji quan, the use of deep abdominal breathing is required; the breath should be deep, long, fine, and even, and be coordinated with body movements. Persistence is important for tai ji quan practice, so persevere and make it a part of your life. After long-term practice, breathing will deepen and the lungs' vital capacity will increase, ensuring a sufficient oxygen supply. When a long-term practitioner is under heavy stress or does physical exercise, his or her body will regulate and deepen breathing spontaneously to ensure there is enough oxygen, without suffering any shortness of breath. Abdominal breathing will enhance diaphragmatic movement and range, and increase the capacity of the chest cavity and negative pressure. This, in turn, promotes blood circulation and metabolism.

Section 4 Effect of Tai Ji Quan on Kidney Function

In traditional Chinese medicine, it is believed that the "waist is the house of the kidney". The kidney has the function of storing essence and regulating lung respiration (i.e., the function of the lung is to receive qi). If there is kidney dysfunction, true yin and true yang will be impaired. This will affect a person's growth, development, and reproductive capabilities, as well as directly affect health and lifespan. If the kidney function in governing qi reception is abnormal, lung respiration will be affected, causing rapid or shallow breathing, and shortness of breath.

During every moment of practice, one should pay special attention to the waist. This will lead to self-massage of the kidneys and increase the kidney's supply of qi and blood. At the same time, the practice of regulating inhalation and exhalation increases the supply of the kidneys' true qi. Together, this will ensure the sufficiency of true yin and true yang, which has the effect of "developing the post-natal essence to supplement the pre-natal". Cultivating qi internally and enhancing its storage is how tai ji quan practice promotes the kidney function of governing qi.

The kidney also "governs bones and generates marrow". The sufficiency of kidney essence is a critical factor in bone strength. Bone growth and development are closely connected to the kidney. Many old people complain that their legs are becoming weaker instead of complaining about growing old. Aging results from the decline of kidney qi, which may manifest as weakness in the lower limbs and other similar symptoms.

When a person is walking, body weight is mainly borne by the lower limbs. The lower limbs need to support two or three times the body weight while walking, and even more so when going up or down stairs. This greatly affects the lower joints. Along with the force of gravity, continued friction between the upper and lower articular surfaces of the knees will damage articular cartilage, narrow joint space, form bone spurs, and sometimes cause joint effusion. These pathological changes are what we usually call the aging of joints, or degenerative arthritis. The pathological changes in the joints can cause so much pain that the patient will be unwilling to move and exercise; muscles will weaken and may even atrophy without sufficient exercise. Weakened muscles will further worsen joint function, resulting in a vicious cycle.

During practice, one must walk like a cat, with footwork that is light, nimble, and steady; empty steps should be clearly distinguished from solid steps. This is excellent training for the lower limbs, especially the knees, bones, muscles, and tendons of the feet. Tai ji quan training correctly targeted at different groups of older people will enhance leg strength, increase stability, and reduce risks of falls and injury. In a study of physical training programs for the elderly in eight treatment centers in the United States, exercises were used that involved endurance, limb extension, and balance training, etc. They were done for different periods of from ten weeks to nine months. Follow-up surveys showed a decrease in falls of 13% for participants over 60 years old, and a decrease of 25% for those over 70. Of all the exercises, the most effective was tai ji quan.

Chapter 5
Characteristics of Different Styles and How to Choose a Style

Section 1 How to Choose a Style as a Beginner

Most tai ji quan practitioners are enthusiastic in the beginning, but without proper guidance and understanding, they tend to mystify it and think it is unfathomable. Some are prejudiced by hearsay, believing there is a rank order among different schools, and that some are better than others. They intently seek a so-called authentic style, and practice routines from just this school, believing all the others are inferior. They are proud to learn this "authentic" style and believe they can attain high level martial skills because they are practicing a "superior" style. Actually, there is no hierarchy of schools and styles. The proper selection of a style should be based on the practitioner's physical condition, personality, talent, and what he or she personally likes instead of on a school's famous reputation. If a young practitioner chooses a slow and soft routine in the beginning, he or she might feel bored. It should be understood that different schools are only different in method, but none of them offer any shortcuts. The undeniable truth for any kind of wu shu is that the practitioner must learn and practice diligently to master martial skills and techniques; there is no exception for anyone or any school.

As we all know, the Chen, Yang, Wú, Wǔ, and Sun styles are the five main schools of tai ji quan, although there are some schools and styles other than the five from which to choose. However, it is better for beginners to learn one of these five main styles since they do not have sufficient knowledge about tai ji quan to tell the difference. They will tend to focus on external movements and postures and not learn true internal martial skills even after some time. Therefore, practitioners should learn one of the five main schools first. Then, after gaining an appreciation for the internal patterns of tai ji quan movement, one may choose to learn one of the other styles. Such a learning process will prevent a practitioner from becoming boastful, sloppy, and undisciplined. The selection of a style should be based on the practitioner's own status and personal preferences. You may first have a look at the routines of different schools and then choose the one you like. Do not think too much about what you can achieve, and do not let other thoughts and ideas distract you from learning and practicing. The five main schools all have long histories, and there are ample reasons why they all have long lineages. It is because they can lead practitioners down the right path without going astray. Looking back on history, great masters have emerged from every one of the five schools. As the saying goes, "All roads lead to Rome." Although the schools all have different approaches, they all aim at the same goal. Success can be assured only with diligent effort, consistent practice and hard work.

To reiterate, the five schools have different characteristics and different teachings which are based on their experiences and understanding. Beginners should select a school which suits them. Learning tai ji quan is a long and slow process. Although there are no shortcuts, proper teaching will make the learning process easier and more enjoyable, and help you to achieve maximum results with less effort. The fame or popularity of a specific school should not be the reason why you choose it. Instead, a beginner should select one according to your own status and preferences. Find a suitable one, practice consistently, and be assured that you will achieve good results with persistent practice. When you gain a deeper understanding after long-term practice, you will then be able to make a wiser choice on whether to continue with the same style or learn another one. Although they are all named tai ji quan schools, each school has different teaching methods and techniques. Each school also has many branches. Study and investigate all of these factors carefully before making your decision.

Although the schools have different teachings, they all share the same ethos and heritage. Although they have different routines and postures, all their movements should be in accordance with the philosophy and principles of tai ji. Although they have different ways of practicing, they can all achieve the same purpose. Each of the different schools has its own body of knowledge and experience, so the choice of a style should be made according to your own likes or dislikes. Success is attainable as long as you are intelligent, healthy and persistent, and you can practice hard and continuously seek self-improvement.

Section 2 Characteristics of Chen Style Tai Ji Quan

Chen style tai ji quan was created by Chen Wang-ting from Chen Jia Gou in Henan Province. It consisted of what we now call, "The Five Chen Style Old Frame Routines." Chen Style was based on the Chen family's art of pugilism, combined with the principles of yin and yang, breathing techniques, *dǎo yǐn* practices from the *Classic of the Yellow Court* (*Huáng Tíng Jīng*, 黄庭经), and combat methods from the *Classic of the Thirty Two Forms of Fist Arts* (*Quán Jīng Sān Shí Èr Shì*, 拳经三十二式) written by Qi Ji-guang. Chen family descendants have transmitted this inheritance to successive generations. Chen style has evolved and two "new frame" routines, arranged in meticulous fashion, were added to the older ones. The new ones are different in speed, intensity, body structure, and application of force compared to the old ones.

Characteristics of Chen Style: In this style, mental consciousness and internal qi movement manifests in the body's external spiral-coiling[8] movement. Chen style emphasizes: using qi to lead and conscious intention to guide movement; maintaining an uplifting energy (*dǐng jìn*, 顶劲) at the vertex of the head; sinking qi to the elixir field, and relaxing and lengthening all the limbs and joints. One should allow the rotation of the hips to lead the rotation of the shoulders and upper and lower limbs, so that the body's spiral-coiling (silk-reeling) movements are integrated; there should be a unity of internal qi movement with external body movement, with all parts linked as one. Chen style is a combination of hardness and softness; the two are complimentary and interdependent. Hardness usually manifests at the end point of a movement, while softness manifests through the movement to the end point. The routines should be performed in a continuous and consistent way without any breaks. Pairs of opposing energies should be unified and coordinated since they are interdependent and inter-transformational; this includes hardness (strength) and softness, opening and closing, fast and slow, bending and straightening, etc. The Chen Style First Routine is comparatively simple, focusing primarily on the use of four of eight energy expressions or techniques: ward-off (*péng*, 掤), yield (*lǚ*, 将), press (*jǐ*, 挤) and push (*àn*, 按); and secondarily on the other four: pluck (*cǎi*, 采), split (*liè*, 挒), elbow (*zhǒu*, 肘), and bump (*kào*, 靠)[9]. Most

---

[8] Spiral-coiling (*chán sī jìn*, 缠丝劲) is also commonly referred to as "*silk reeling*".
[9] 掤、捋、挤、按、采、挒、肘、靠

movements should be soft; in the midst of softness, there is hardness; softness should temper hardness. Use conscious intention to move qi, and use qi to drive body movement. The focus is primarily on the training of spiral-coiling (silk-reeling) energy and only secondarily on the emission of power (*fā jìn*). Soft coiling movements that are slow and steady characterize this routine. External and internal, movement and stillness are in harmony; a slight movement in one part of the body activates movement of the entire body. The Chen Style Second Routine is much more complicated, focusing primarily on the techniques: pluck, split, elbow and bump; and secondarily on ward-off, yield, press and push. This routine is fast with tightly knit movements. There is more hardness and less softness, and there is softness within hardness, which implies softness through strength. Its primary emphasis is on hard force, which includes shaking, foot stomping, leaping, jumping, and sudden weight shifts. Spiral-coiling (silk-reeling) movements in this routine should be strong, fast and crisp.

Key Points of Chen Style Body Mechanics: Use conscious intention to move qi. The waist originates all movement. Rotate the waist to drive the rotation of the trunk and the movement of every other part of the body. Other key points include relaxation, flexibility, elasticity, shaking force, spiral-coiling (silk-reeling) energy, and foot stomping to initiate force.

Section 3 Characteristics of Yang Style Tai Ji Quan

Yang Style was created by Yang Fu-kui[10] (also known as Yang Lu-chan[11]) from Yong Nian County in Hebei Province. He learned Chen style tai ji quan from Chen Chang-xing during the Qing Dynasty's Dao Guang period, then went to Beijing to teach tai ji quan in 1850.

To better meet the healthcare needs of high-ranking officials, the wealthy, and the elderly, as well as those with weaker physical constitutions, Yang Fu-kui started to modify the Chen style. He deleted power emission (*fā jìn*) and forceful movements such as foot stomping, jumping, and leaping from the Chen style old frame routines, and eventually created the structure of the Yang Style. The creation of the Yang style increased the popularity of tai ji quan and broadened its appeal. Later, it was modified by Yang Jian-hou into a middle frame routine, and then further modified by Yang Cheng-fu intoa, large frame routine, which became the Yang style we practice today.

Characteristics of Yang Style: The style's movements are graceful and extended, simple but tightly arranged. Footwork is light and nimble, but steady. The body structure is upright. It has both hardness and softness, with movements that are smooth and fluid, simple to learn and practice. During practice, the body is relaxed and comfortable. With relaxation comes softness; increased softness produces strength; the two reinforce each other to create one. As Yang Cheng-fu said, tai ji quan is "a needle concealed in cotton," an art of strength expressed in the form of softness.

Key Points of Yang Style Body Mechanics: Yang Cheng-fu summarized Yang style body mechanics into ten techniques or requirements:

(1) Suspend and lift the vertex of the head (虚灵顶劲)

(2) Relax the chest and round the back (含胸拔背)

(3) Relax the waist (松腰)

---

[10] 杨福魁

[11] 杨露禅 , Yang Fu-kui's courtesy name

(4) Distinguish empty and solid movements (分虚实)

(5) Sink the shoulders and drop the elbows (沈肩坠肘)

(6) Use conscious intention (*yì*, 意) instead of force (*lì*, 力) (用意不用力)

(7) Coordinate the upper and lower body (上下相随)

(8) Integrate the interior and exterior of the body (内外相合)

(9) Link movements without any breaks (相连不断)

(10) Seek stillness in motion (动中求静)

Section 4 Characteristics of Wǔ Style Tai Ji Quan

Wǔ Style was created by Wu Yu-xiang from Yong Nian County in Hebei Province. Wu Yu-xiang started learning wu shu as well as literature as a child. He studied under Yang Lu-chan in 1850 and learned the Chen style old frame routine. In 1852, he passed through Zhao Bao township in Henan Province and learned the Chen style new frame routine from Chen Qing-ping. After that, Wu Yu-xiang intensively studied the principles and structures of tai ji quan, became more knowledgeable, and subsequently created Wǔ style tai ji quan. Although this style was based on the Chen and Yang styles, it is different from both schools and has its own unique flavor.

Characteristics of Wǔ Style: The movements are simple but compactly arranged. The body postures are stable; the left and right hands are responsible for movements of the left and right sides of the body, respectively, with no overlap. The movements of the hands should not go beyond the toes, and should stick close to the body trunk when retracting. The postural structure is small but not constrained; the movements are slow and soft, and the body is straight and upright. The trunk should maintain central equilibrium, whether the body is rotating, advancing, or retreating. There are strict requirements about footwork. Practitioners must distinguish empty from solid. The steps are light and nimble; place the foot on the ground gradually, with the toes touching the ground first and then the heel. The knee of the front leg should not go beyond the toes in a bow stance, and the back leg should stay low. Movements should be fluid and smooth, emphasizing "initiation, continuity, opening, and closing." One should integrate external physical movement with the dynamics of internal qi movement. Contain the mind and consciousness; lead qi movement with conscious intention, and lead body movement with qi movement. The aim is to achieve of unity of conscious intention (*yì*), qi, and force (*lì*), with all three inseparable. In such a state, the qi and body will move together and follow conscious intention, and the qi and force will go wherever intention goes.

Key Points of Wǔ Style Body Mechanics: Relax the chest and round the back; retract the hips and buttocks; suspend the vertex; protect and suspend the crotch; drop the elbows; and align the tailbone.

Section 5 Characteristics of Wú Style Tai Ji Quan

Wu Jian-quan was a native from Da Xing in Hebei Province. His father, Quan-you, learned tai ji quan from Yang Lu-chan when Yang was teaching tai ji quan in Beijing; he then learned from Yang Ban-hou, the second son of Yang Lu-chan. Quan-you gradually modified the small frame routine from the Yang style. Wu Jian-quan made further changes and eventually created Wú style tai ji quan.

Characteristics of Wú Style: Wú style is characterized by gentleness and is well-known for being able to transform force. It has a serene and natural flavor; the movements are light, gentle, fluid, and done without breaks in momentum. It has a peaceful quality. The structure is compact and small, but not constrained. Since it is based on the foundation of the large frame routine, the movements are extended. The toes of both feet should point forward in the bow stance, and the vertex of the head should form a diagonal with the heel of the back foot. In horse stance, body weight should be loaded more on either the left or right, whichever is the attack side. When turning the body to change direction, no matter 45, 90 or 180 degrees, the whole foot should roll and turn.

Key Points of Wú Style Body Mechanics: Suspend the vertex of the head and relax the neck; relax the chest and round the back; rotate and spiral the wrists and shoulders; spread the fingers and stretch open the palms; bow the waist, retract the buttocks, and bend the knees and sink the body.

Section 6 Characteristics of Sun Style Tai Ji Quan

Sun style was created by Sun Lu-tang from Wan County in Hebei Province. He learned Wú style from Hao Wei-zhen shortly after China became a republic. Based on the Wú style, Sun combined the advancing and retreating steps from *xíng yì quán*, and the nimble twisting and turning body movements of *bā guà zhǎng*. With a comprehensive understanding of these different styles, Sun combined the two with tai ji quan to create the Sun style.

Characteristics of Sun Style: The postures are high, and the footwork soft, slow, and smooth. The movements are small, light, and nimble, with one foot following the other; there are a variety of directional changes. When advancing, the back leg follows the front leg as it steps forward; when retreating, the front leg follows the back leg as it steps backward. Sun Style is called the "tai ji quan of flexible steps." The routine's basic transitions and coordinated movements are linked by "hands opening" and "hands closing" techniques; thus, Sun style is also called the "tai ji quan of opening and closing". Movements are extended, smooth, flexible, nimble, and natural. Empty steps are distinguished from solid steps; the movements are as fluid as flowing water and floating clouds, and every turn and rotation of the body are connected by "opening" and "closing" movements; therefore, it is also called the "tai ji quan of opening and closing and flexible steps".

Key Points of Sun Style Body Mechanics: The feet follow each other, with the back leg following the front to step forward, while the front leg follows the back leg to step back. Empty and solid steps should be clearly distinguished. The style's characteristic opening and closing movements connect the entire routine.

Chapter 6
Basic Postures and Requirements of Tai Ji Quan

Section 1 Basic Postures of Tai Ji Quan

1. Basic Hand Formations

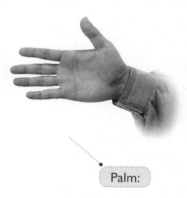

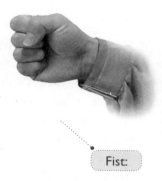

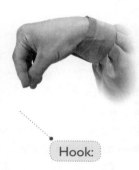

Palm:

Fist:

Hook:

Open the hand, separate and bend the five fingers slightly, relax and do not over-extend the palm; keep the shape of the "tiger's mouth" (the junction between the thumb and index finger) round and smooth.

Relax the four fingers and roll them together toward the center of the palm; press the thumb lightly against the second joints of the index finger and middle finger.

Join all the fingers together and bend the wrist.

2. Basic Body Postures

Natural Posture:

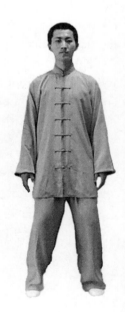

Stand with the feet parallel and shoulder-width apart, with toes pointing forward. Bend the knees slightly, but not beyond the toes. Touch the upper palate with the tip of the tongue. Imagine that the vertex of the head—DU 20 (*bǎi huì*, 百会)—is on a vertical line with the perineum (*huì yīn*, 会阴), and push the vertex upward as if it were suspended. Straighten the neck, and pull the chin in slightly. Sink (relax) the chest, and sink the qi to the elixir field. Relax the waist and position the buttocks as if you were starting to sit down. Keep the curvature of the spine as straight as possible, sinking the weight of each vertebra, one by one, toward the center of the soles. Do not press the arms against the trunk of the body, and keep a hollow space under the armpits. Relax and sink the shoulders, drop the arms and slightly turn the elbows outward. Let the arms hang loosely beside the body. The eyes gaze horizontally forward.

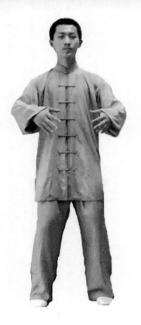

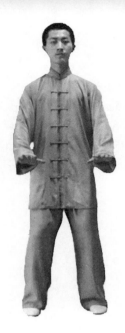

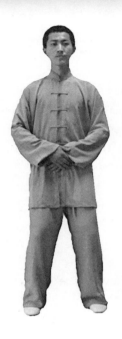

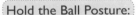

Hold the Ball Posture:

Stand in a Natural Posture and position the arms in front of the abdomen as if holding a large ball. The joints of the upper limbs should appear rounded, not angular. Close the eyes slightly and gaze downward 45 degrees to the front.

Pressing Posture:

Stand in a Natural Posture, and press the hands down in front of the thighs, with fingers pointing forward. Do not allow the arms to press against the body and keep a hollow space under the armpits; sink the shoulders and drop the elbows.

Hands Overlapping Posture:

Stand in a Natural Posture, overlap the hands and press the abdomen; place the center of the palms—PC 8 (*láo gōng*, 劳宫)—on top of the navel or right under the navel.

3. Basic Footwork

Ready Posture 预备式

(1) Stand with the feet together, and let the arms hang loosely alongside the body. Straighten the neck, suspend the vertex, regulate the breath, and gaze horizontally forward.

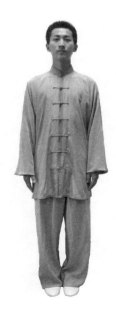

Opening 开步

(2) Shift the weight to the right leg, move the left foot a half step to the left, then distribute the weight evenly between both legs. Keep the point KI 1 (*yǒng quán*, 涌泉) on the feet positioned vertically below the two GB 21 (*jiān jǐng*, 肩井) points on shoulders. Eyes gaze horizontally forward.

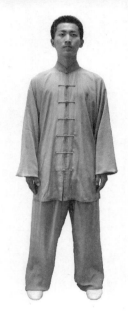

Left Bow Stance 左弓步

(3) Rotate the waist slightly leftward and shift the weight to the left leg as the waist rotates. At the same time, rotate the right foot inward by pivoting on the heel and turning the toes 45 degrees to the left front; bend the arms slightly, and look horizontally forward.

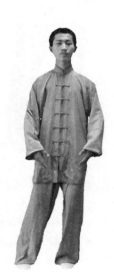

(4) Rotate the waist slightly leftward, and shift all the weight to the right leg. Move the left foot to the medial side of the right foot, with toes lightly touching the ground. Withdraw the hands and overlap them on the abdomen, pointing the fingers 45 degrees downward. The eyes gaze horizontally forward.

(5) Rotate the waist slightly leftward, and step the left foot forward to the left; the heel makes light contact with the ground. The eyes gaze horizontally forward.

(6) Plant the left foot solidly on the ground and shift the body weight forward to form a left bow stance. The eyes gaze horizontally forward.

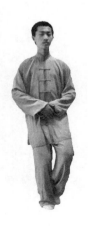

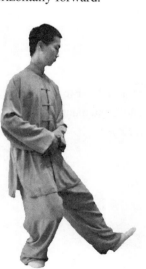

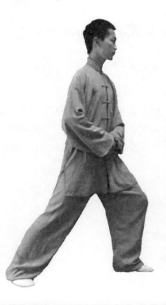

Right Bow Stance 右弓步

(7) Rotate the waist leftward, and turn the front foot outward 45 degrees by pivoting on the heel. Root the weight on the feet and shift the weight forward. Then, lift the right heel. The eyes gaze horizontally forward.

(8) Continue to rotate the waist leftward until all the weight is on the left leg. Draw the right foot to the medial side of the left foot, with the toes lightly contacting the ground; eyes gaze horizontally forward.

(9) Rotate the waist slightly rightward, and step the right foot forward to the right; the heel lightly contacts the ground. The eyes gaze horizontally forward.

(10) Plant the front foot solidly on the ground, and shift the body weight forward to form a right bow stance. The eyes gaze horizontally forward.

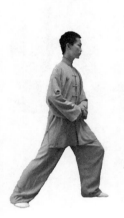 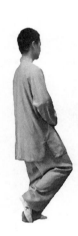 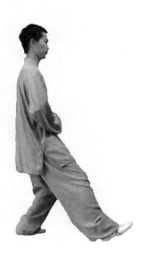 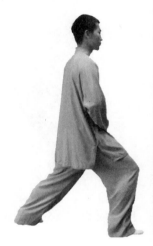

Left Bow Stance 左弓步

(11) Turn the waist rightward, and rotate the front foot outward by pivoting on the heel and turning the toes 45 degrees to the right. Root the weight on the feet and then shift it forward while lifting the left heel. The eyes gaze horizontally forward.

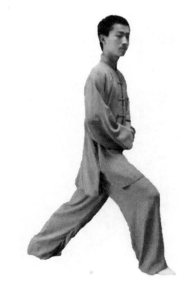

(12) Rotate the waist slightly rightward, and move the body slowly forward to the right. Draw the left foot to the medial side of the right foot; the ball of the foot lightly contacts the ground. The eyes gaze horizontally forward.

(13) Rotate the waist slightly leftward, and step the left foot forward to the left; the heel lightly contacts the ground. The eyes gaze horizontally forward.

(14) Plant the left foot solidly on the ground, then shift the body weight forward to form a left bow stance. The eyes gaze horizontally forward.

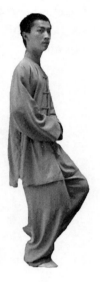 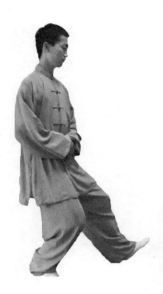 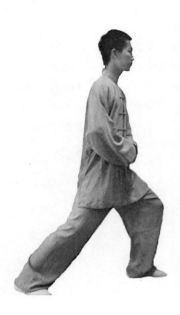

Turning the Body   转身

(15) Shift the weight backward to the right foot and lift the left toes. The eyes gaze horizontally forward.

(16) Rotate the waist right, and turn the left foot inward 120 degrees by pivoting on the heel. The eyes gaze horizontally forward.

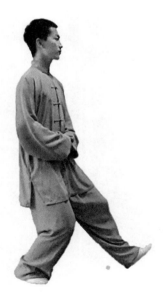 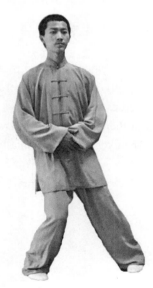

Right Bow Stance 变右弓步

(17) Continue to rotate the waist rightward and shift the body weight backward to the left leg. Draw the right foot to the medial side of the left foot. The ball of the right foot makes light contact with the ground. The eyes gaze horizontally forward.

(18) Rotate the waist rightward and step the right foot forward to the right; the heel lightly contacts the ground. The eyes gaze horizontally forward.

(19) Plant the right foot solidly on the ground and shift the body weight forward to form a right bow stance. The eyes gaze horizontally forward.

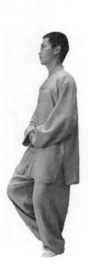 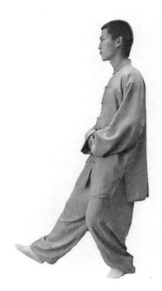 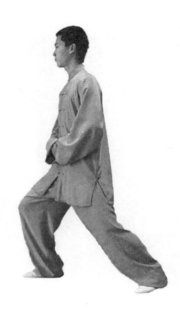

Repeat the left and right bow steps once each and form a right bow stance at the end. The eyes gaze horizontally forward.

Feet Together 合步

(20) Shift the body weight to the left leg and lift the right toes. The eyes gaze horizontally forward.

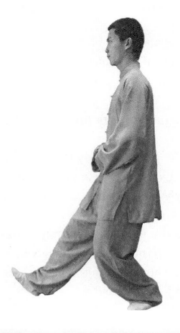

(21) Rotate the waist leftward, and turn the right foot inward by pivoting on the heel; point the toes in the same direction as in the Opening Posture. The eyes gaze horizontally forward.

(22) Shift the body weight to the right leg and lift the left heel; the toes lightly contact the ground. The eyes gaze horizontally forward.

(23) Draw the left foot back together with the right foot, planting it solidly on the ground; then, shift the weight so that it is distributed evenly between both legs. Straighten the legs slowly while relaxing; drop the hands alongside the body. The eyes gaze horizontally forward.

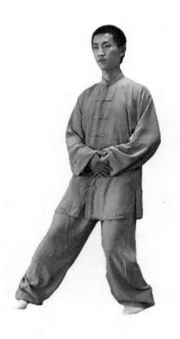
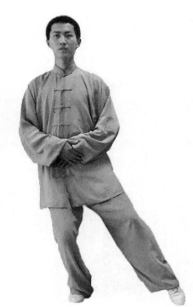
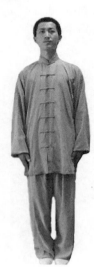

Section 2 Basic Requirements for Tai Ji Quan Practice

Regulation of body movements, regulation of breath, and regulation of mind are the three essential elements of tai ji quan; the basic requirements for tai ji quan practice are mainly focused on these three elements.

1. Requirements for Body Movements

❂ Correct Body Posture

"*Qi cannot flow smoothly if the posture is incorrect; the mind will be restless if qi cannot flow smoothly; spirit will be scattered if the mind is restless* (形不正则气不顺,气不顺则意不宁,意不宁则神散乱)." The aim of tai ji quan practice is to achieve a healthy state with free and smooth respiration, a peaceful mind, and a comfortable body. Breathing and the channels and collaterals are all connected to body posture; poor posture will lead to an uncomfortable feeling caused by the obstruction of qi and blood. This will result in listlessness and fatigue. Therefore, proper body posture is a basic requirement for tai ji quan practice.

To achieve correct posture, one must know the starting and ending points of the movements, as well as the transitions from one point to the next, and their overall effect on posture and movement. Conscious intention should guide hand positions and gestures, stepping patterns, and footwork to meet specifications. However, they should be done in a natural, relaxed manner; the movements should be accurate, coherent, and fluid. The upper body should be light and nimble, and the lower body steady and solid, so as to establish a foundation for relaxation, peace and naturalness.

☯ Relaxation, Peace and Naturalness

"Relaxation" is achieved from exterior to interior, and also from interior to exterior. Correct posture is formed by lengthening (loosening) the joints, and allowing the body's structure to stretch naturally. It requires letting the mind become free, easy, and comfortable. Relaxation is different from laxity. In a state of relaxation, the joints are lengthened while body movements are flexible and fluid, with changes and transitions made as the mind dictates. As for laxity, the joints are constricted and movements are slack and lack strength; the body cannot move as you intend, and the mind is fatigued and without spirit. The state of "peace" is achieved by keeping out all distractions during practice and is based on relaxation. "Naturalness" is based on relaxation and peace; it means that during practice one should not be overly intent on achieving results.

☯ Waist is the Key for All Movements

The waist is the key that connects all the movements and changes in tai ji quan practice. That is to say, the waist and spine are the axis of rotation that links all movements and transformations. The waist is the junction between the upper and lower body, the central pivot that allows the limbs to move flexibly, and the gateway that leads to the unity of body and mind. Therefore, by controlling the waist, one has grasped a key tai ji quan principle.

The technique of controlling the waist involves relaxing the waist and restraining the buttocks (retracting the coccyx slightly so that it does not stick out). When performing a movement, relax the waist and retract the buttocks. At the same time, relax and sink the weight of each vertebra, one by one, and the body weight onto the feet. A key point in the application of force is that it is initiated by the spine, controlled by the waist, rooted in the feet, and expressed in the fingers. The sequential flow for the upper limbs starts at the tip section (i.e., fingers), followed by the middle section (i.e., elbows), and is activated by the root section (i.e., shoulders). On the lower limbs, it is initiated by the root section (i.e., hips), flows to the middle section (i.e., knees), and reaches the end section (toes). The movements of the upper and lower body should be coordinated, with force transmitted throughout the entire body so that it reaches the limbs, fingers, and toes.

☯ Smooth, Flexible, and Coherent

Body postures should appear round and smooth, forming full arcs in the movements. The movements must not be stiff or rigid, but should be flexible and nimble and follow one's intentions. They should be performed at an even and consistent pace without any breaks or obvious changes in height. Movements should be fluid, soft, and steady like flowing water and floating clouds. The key to being smooth, flexible, and coherent is to use the waist as the axis for all movements.

2. Requirements for the Mind

Focus the mind and allow the spirit to be at ease and comfortable during practice; this is achieved from a state of relaxation, peace, and naturalness.

☯ Correct Physical Structure

Tai ji quan beginners are usually not used to the form and structure of the movements; they do not yet have sufficient control of their muscles, and thus will easily lose their postural structure. Therefore, they should focus their mind on the correct specifications required for each movement. This will prevent any discomfort caused by the non-smooth flow of qi and blood that results from improper body structure and movement.

☯ Faintly Discernible

For those who are already familiar with the movements, they are able to relax their bodies naturally, and can achieve an easy and comfortable state of mind. This is a state of high concentration with no distracting thoughts. The qi in the channels and collaterals will be activated gradually, and flow smoothly along specific routes according to the body's pugilistic movements. This process combines with the "strength (*li*)" produced by muscle contraction to form "power (*jìn*)." The flow of qi follows the mind's intention. The more relaxed the mind is, the more steady and more substantial the force becomes, and the efficiency will increase as a result. In contrast, if the mind is tense or has distracting thoughts, the circulation of qi and blood will be affected, the force will be weakened, and efficiency will decrease. The level of force is a criterion for evaluating the level of the practitioner. Therefore, keep out distractions as much as possible and reduce mental activities to a faintly discernible level.

3. Requirements for the Breath

(1) Breath regulation is the basis of relaxation, peace, and naturalness. Breathing is a form of physical movement—the contraction of the diaphragm relies on the relaxation of the body and a peaceful mind.

(2) Do not intentionally try to force yourself to breath in any specific way. Breathing should be a natural reflection of a physical and mental state of peace and relaxation. Trying too hard to breath in a certain way may cause uncomfortable symptoms, including chest discomfort and mental stress.

(3) Body movements and breathing should be synchronized. Inhalation usually accompanies opening and ascending movements, and exhalation is usually done with closing and descending movements.

There are three common breathing techniques used in tai ji quan practice, but all of them should be done in a natural and relaxed way.

☯ Natural Breathing

This is same as the type of breathing one uses in daily life without conscious effort, and there is no need to make any obvious adjustments. This is the preliminary breathing technique used in tai ji quan practice. As you enhance your martial skills, you will naturally adapt to the two other breathing techniques described below and gradually be able to achieve unity of body, qi, and mind.

☯ Abdominal Breathing

The abdomen expands or contracts while breathing. This breathing technique helps focus the mind and improves internal organ function. There are two kinds of abdominal breathing:

(1) Regular Abdominal Breathing: The abdomen expands while inhaling, and returns to its normal position while exhaling.

(2) Reverse Abdominal Breathing: The abdomen contracts while inhaling, and returns to its normal position while exhaling.

Section 3 Common Problems and Solutions Found in Teaching Tai Ji Quan

1. Inability to Relax: Causes and Solutions

(1) Tension in the body caused by improper movement and posture

Solution: Try to understand thoroughly the key points and sequences of all the postures, movements, transitions, and weight shifts; then try to experience the feeling of being relaxed and free of excess tension as you practice.

(2) Tension in the body caused by trying too hard to "relax" or trying too hard to regulate "breathing"

Solution: Everything requires persistence, but you must proceed step by step, realizing that "haste only makes waste". During practice, relax and remember the principle of "naturalness", and the tension caused by trying too hard will disappear.

(3) Tension in the body caused by certain diseases

Solution: While warming up, self-massage problem areas or where there is discomfort, freeing the flow of qi and blood. Be cautious and adjust the intensity of practice to prevent mistakes.

(4) Tension of the body caused by insufficient warm-up exercises

Solution: Before performing the routine, do some simple stretching and warm-up exercises. This will help loosen joints, relax muscles, and circulate qi and blood.

2. Inability to Concentrate: Causes and Solutions

(1) Lack of confidence

Solution: Nothing is too difficult for those who try, so be confident and use confidence as a foundation to shape your thinking.

(2) Improper understanding of techniques and key points
Solution: Let your practice be based on an understanding of the principles and key points.

(3) Personal qualities
Solution: Enhance self-cultivation, and try to achieve a peaceful and calm physical and emotional state in daily life. Train yourself to be more tolerant and not be disturbed by negative events and negative emotions.

(4) Environmental factors
Solution: Choose either a quiet indoor or outdoor environment when you practice, avoiding drafts or windy conditions; the temperature should be comfortable, and there should be gentle lighting and fresh air.

(5) Unpredictable factors
Solution: Do not force yourself to practice if you suffer from mood swings or feel emotionally unstable, or just cannot concentrate no matter how much you try.

Chapter 7
Yang Style 40 Movements Tai Ji Quan Routine

Ready Posture 预备势

1. Stand with feet together facing south, suspend the head with energy going up to the vertex, and pull the chin in slightly. Relax the entire body, contain the mind and regulate the breath.

2. Shift the weight slowly to the right leg, and lift the left foot slowly.

3. Step the left foot to the left so that the feet are shoulder-width apart, with toes pointing forward; feet adhere effortlessly to the ground. Body weight is distributed evenly over both legs, arms hang loosely on the sides, and eyes gaze horizontally forward.

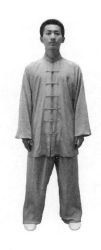

Movement 1: Opening 起势

1. Slowly raise the arms up in front to shoulder-height; keep the arms shoulder-width apart, with palms facing downward.

2. Sink the shoulders and drop the elbows; press the palms downward until they are in front of the thighs. The fingers point forward and eyes gaze horizontally forward.

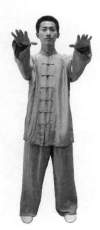

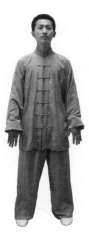

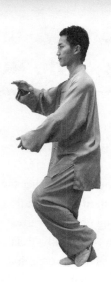

Movement 2a: Step Forward & Ward Off 上步掤

1. Rotate the waist rightward, turn the right toes outward 45 degrees, and then shift the weight to the right leg; then, draw the left foot back to the medial side of the right foot. At the same time, rotate the right palm so that it faces down and raise it in front of the chest. Simultaneously, move the left palm in front of the abdomen, facing up; the palms face each other and the eyes gaze horizontally at the right front.

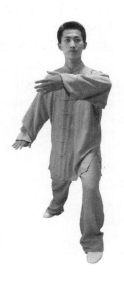

2. Slowly step the left foot forward to the left front, first touching the heel on the ground lightly. Then, slowly shift the weight forward so that the left foot is solidly planted on the ground to form a left bow stance[12]. Next, rotate the waist slightly to the right while shifting the body weight forward. At the same time, move the left arm to the left front to ward-off (*péng*); the left arm forms a curved arc with the palm facing inward. Press the right palm down near the right hip, keeping it a fist's distance away from the body. The eyes gaze horizontally at the right front.

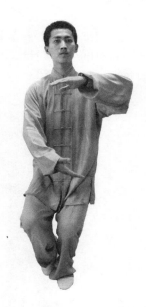

Movement 2b: Grasp the Sparrow's Tail 揽雀尾

1. Shift the body weight slowly to the left foot, drawing the right foot back to the medial side of the left foot; at the same time, rotate the waist slightly leftward while rotating the left arm so that the palm faces down in front of the chest. Simultaneously, rotate the right arm with palm facing up in front of the abdomen; the palms face each other, and eyes gaze horizontally at the left front.

---

[12] In the bow stance, the front leg is bent at the knee and bears about 70% of the body weight, while the rear leg is straight and bears about 30%.

2. Step the right leg forward to the right; the heel lightly contacts the ground as weight shifts to the right leg to form a solid right bow stance. At the same time, rotate the waist rightward, and move the right arm to ward-off (*péng*); the right arm is curved and forms an arc with the palm facing inward at chest level. Simultaneously, press the left palm, which faces down and is level, next to the left hip. The eyes gaze horizontally forward.

3. Rotate the waist rightward while moving the right arm to the right; the arm rotates inward (clockwise) as it extends forward. At the same time, rotate the left palm outward (counterclockwise) and move it rightward next to the medial side of the right elbow. The eyes gaze horizontally toward the right hand. Next, shift the weight backward, rotating the waist leftward. At the same time, both palms follow the weight shift and deflect back (*lǚ*) to the left rear; the hands are about level with the abdomen; eyes look at the right hand.

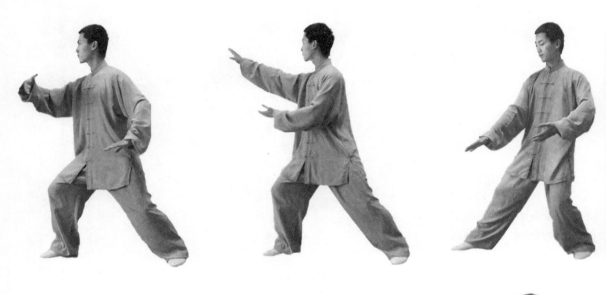

4. Rotate the waist slightly leftward while raising both arms; they overlap in front of the chest to form an arc, with the left palm facing outward and the right palm inward. Rotate the waist rightward as you shift the body weight to the right to form a right bow stance. Then press (*jǐ*) the arms forward to the right front at chest height. The eyes gaze horizontally forward.

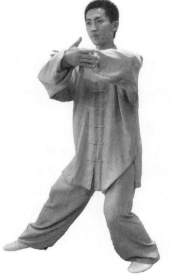

5. Rotate the arms so that the palms face down and extend them forward; they should be at the same height and shoulder-width apart; the eyes look at the hands. Then, shift the weight backward, drawing the palms back down in front of the abdomen; face the palms to the lower front; eyes look forward at the hands.

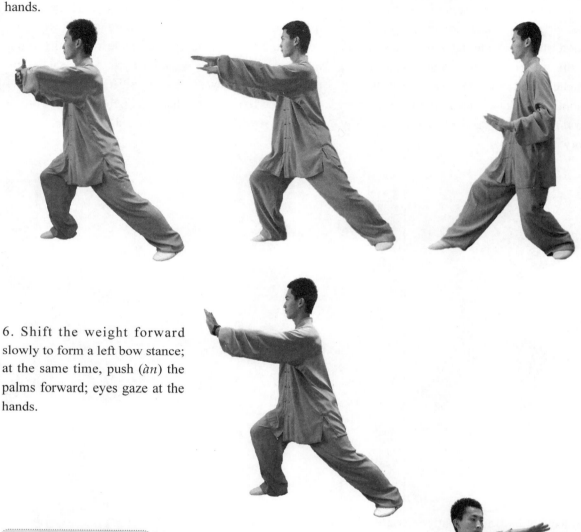

6. Shift the weight forward slowly to form a left bow stance; at the same time, push (*àn*) the palms forward; eyes gaze at the hands.

Movement 3: Single Whip 单鞭

1. Rotate the waist leftward, shift the body weight slowly to the left leg, and turn the right toes inward 45 degrees. At same time, move the palms slowly and horizontally to the left side of the body, with palms facing down at the same height and shoulder-width apart. The eyes gaze horizontally at the left front.

2. Rotate the waist rightward, and move the hands inward, then outward and finally to the right side of the body. Shift the weight slowly to the right leg, draw the left foot back to the medial side of the right foot; at the same time, join the fingers of the right hand and bend the wrist to form a hook. As the waist rotates, move the left palm to the medial side of the right arm; eyes gaze at the right hook.

3. Rotate the waist leftward, and step the left foot to the left front; the heel first touches the ground lightly as the body weight shifts forward, then the foot is planted solidly to form a left bow stance. Simultaneously, the left palm follows the rotation of the waist and moves to the left side of the body before it pushes forward. The eyes gaze at the left palm.

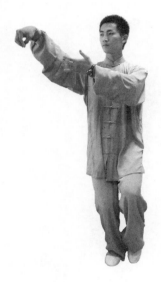

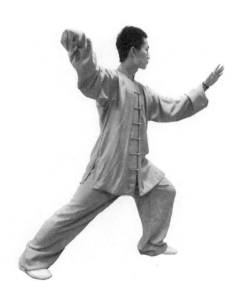

| Movement 4: Raise Hands & Step Forward | 提手上势

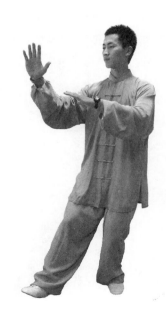

Shift the weight backward to the right leg as the waist rotates to the right; at the same time, turn the left foot inward 45 degrees. Then, shift the weight to the left leg and draw the palms back in front of the chest. Step the right foot a half step forward and to the right to form a right empty stance; the heel lightly contacts the ground while the palms push forward slightly. The left and right palms are at chest and shoulder level, respectively; the right palm faces left, and the left palm faces right; the fingers point diagonally upward. The eyes gaze horizontally at the right palm.

Movement 5: White Crane Spreads Wings　白鹤亮翅

1. Rotate the waist leftward and turn the right foot inward 120 degrees; drop the right arm in a curve diagonally to the left in front of the abdomen, with palm facing up. At the same time, rotate the left arm so that the palm faces down and move it in front of the chest; the palms face each other.

2. Rotate the waist rightward and shift all the body weight to the right leg while drawing the left foot back to the medial side of the right foot; the left toes lightly contact the ground to form a left empty stance. Raise both arms to the right in a curved line diagonally to the right above the head; face the right palm forward and move the left hand next to the medial side of the right forearm.

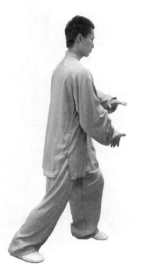
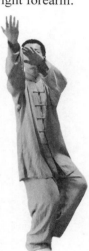

3. Rotate the waist leftward, and step the left foot half a step forward as the waist rotates; the toes lightly touch the ground to form a left empty stance. At the same time, drop the left hand to the lower left. The base of the left palm is beside the left hip and is the locus of force (*li*) for the hand; the fingers point forward. The eyes gaze horizontally forward.

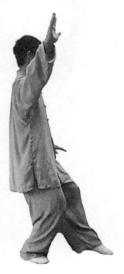
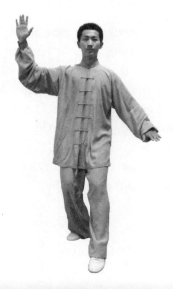

Movement 6: Twist Step & Brush Knee 搂膝拗步

1. Rotate the waist leftward slightly while moving the right arm forward to shoulder-height. Then, rotate the waist rightward and move the right arm rearward passing the right hip, and angle the palm diagonally upward as you move it above the right shoulder. As the waist rotates, move the left palm past the chest and then in front of the right shoulder. At the same time, shift all the weight to the right leg and draw the left foot back to the medial side of the right foot; the right toes lightly touch the ground. The eyes gaze horizontally at the right palm.

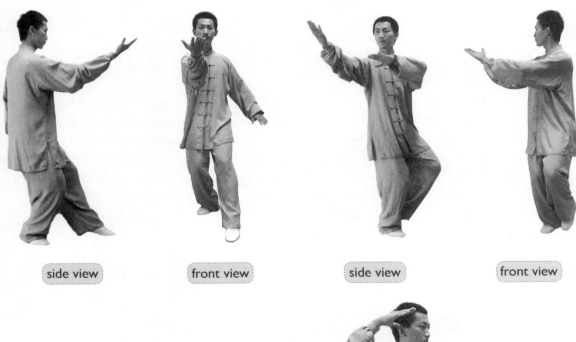

side view   front view   side view   front view

2. Step the left foot forward to the left front, lightly touching the heel on the ground, while moving the left hand in front of the chest; at the same time, draw the right hand beside the right ear with the palm facing inward.

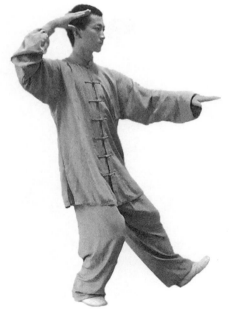

3. Slowly shift the weight forward, transferring the weight to the front foot to form a left bow stance. At the same time, rotate the waist leftward and press the left palm downward in front of the left hip with fingers pointing forward. Simultaneously, push the right palm forward; the base of palm should be level. The eyes gaze at the right hand.

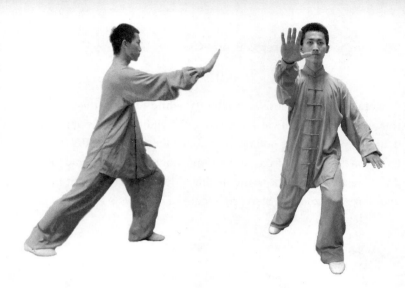

4. Rotate the waist leftward and turn the toes outward 45 degrees, shifting the body weight slowly to the left leg; draw the right foot to the medial side of the left foot with toes touching the ground lightly. At the same time, rotate the left arm and move it diagonally to the left rear in a curved line until it is about shoulder-height. Simultaneously, move the right hand to the medial side of the left elbow, palm facing down; eyes gaze horizontally at the left palm.

5. Rotate the waist rightward, stepping the right foot forward and to the right front; lightly touch the heel on the ground. Draw the left hand to beside the left ear with the palm facing inward, and move the right palm to the front of the body.

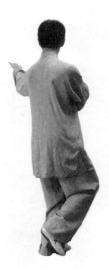

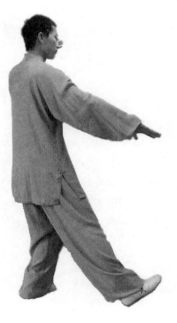

6. Slowly shift the body weight forward, stepping the front foot solidly on the ground to form a right bow stance. At the same time, rotate the waist right, pressing the right palm downward and to the right so that it is next to the right hip, with fingers pointing forward. Simultaneously, push the left palm forward; the base of palm should be shoulder-level. The eyes gaze at the left hand.

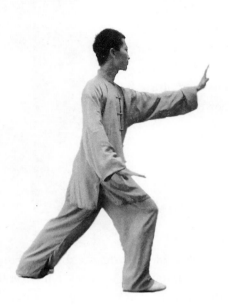
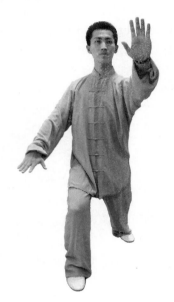

7. Rotate the waist rightward and turn the right toes outward 45 degrees, and then shift the weight slowly to the right leg while drawing the left foot back to the medial side of the right foot, with the toes lightly touching the ground. At the same time, rotate the right arm diagonally backward in a curved line to the right rear until it is level with the shoulders. Simultaneously, move the left palm to the medial side of the right elbow, palm facing down; eyes gaze horizontally at the right hand.

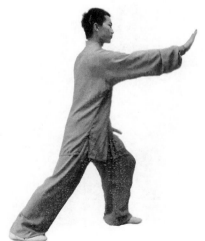

8. Same as step 2 of this movement.

Movement 7: Hands Strum the Lute   手揮琵琶

Slowly shift the body weight forward to the left leg, and slowly step the right foot forward for a half step behind the left leg; then, shift the weight back to the right leg and lift the left toes, with the heel lightly touching the ground to form a left empty stance. At the same time, rotate the waist slightly rightward and raise the left palm upward, with fingers at nose-level. Simultaneously, draw the right palm back to the medial side of the left elbow; eyes gaze horizontally at the left index finger.

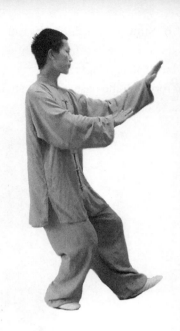

Movement 8: Parry & Punch   搬拦捶

1. Rotate the waist left, turn the left toes outward 45 degrees, then shift all the weight to the left leg; draw the right foot back to the medial side of the left foot, lightly touching the toes to the ground. At the same time, move the left palm in front of the chest with the palm facing inward; change the right palm to a fist and drop it in front of the abdomen.

2. Rotate the waist rightward, and step the right foot forward, touching the heel lightly on the ground; then, slowly shift the weight forward, planting the foot solidly on the ground to form a right bow stance. As the waist rotates, move the right fist in an arc as it deflects forward and downward while passing the chest; protect the medial side of the right elbow with the left palm.

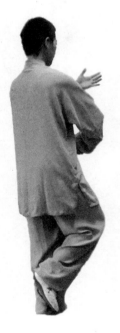 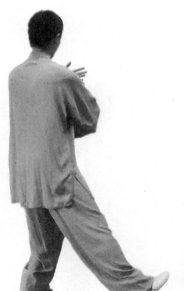 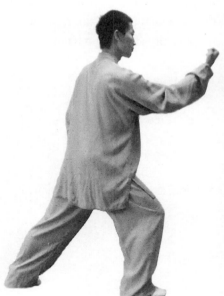

3. Continue rotating the waist rightward while turning the right toes outward 45 degrees. Slowly shift the body weight back onto the right foot, and lift the left heel and draw it to the medial side of the right foot. At the same time, extend the left arm forward slowly while moving the right arm rearward to the right side of the body at chest-level; eyes gaze at the right fist.

4. Rotate the waist slightly rightward, and step the left foot forward with the heel lightly touching the ground. Draw the right fist back beside the right hip. Simultaneously, move the left palm in front of the body to parry (*lán*, 拦); the palm is chest-level and faces the lower right front.

5. Rotate the waist leftward, slowly shift the body weight forward and plant the front foot solidly on the ground to form a left bow stance. The right fist punches forward with the eye of the fist[13] facing up at chest-height; protect the medial side of the right elbow with the left palm facing right; eyes gaze horizontally at the right fist.

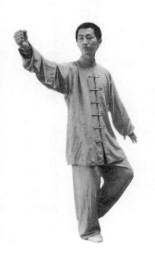 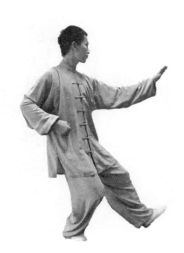 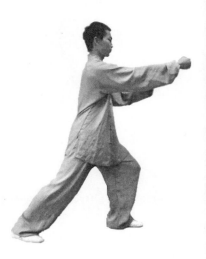

Movement 9: Apparent Close 如封四闭

1. Move the left hand across and under the right elbow, and then extend it forward. Change the right fist to a palm and rotate both wrists so that they face upward.

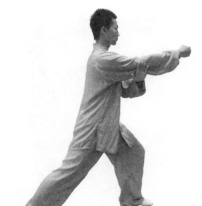 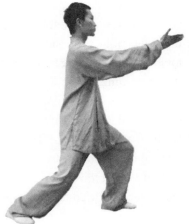

---

[13] Eye of the fist is the area located between the thumb and index finger.

2. Shift the weight back onto the right leg and rotate the waist slightly rightward, drawing the palms back toward the abdomen with the palms facing down.

3. Shift the weight forward to form a left bow stance. At the same time, rotate the waist slightly leftward, pushing the palms forward; fingers point upward with the base of palm at shoulder-level; eyes gaze horizontally at the hands.

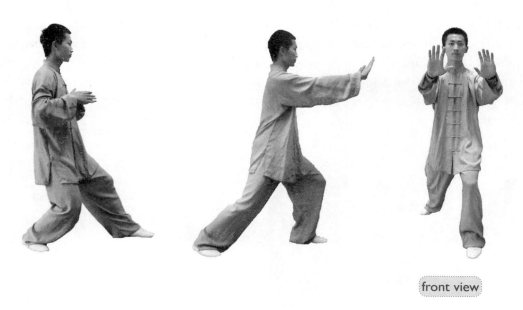

front view

Movement 10: Diagonal Flying　斜飞势

1. Rotate the waist rightward, shift the weight to the right leg and turn the left toes inward and to the right 120 degrees; rotate the waist leftward, and shift the weight slowly to the left leg, then draw the right foot back to the medial side of the left foot. At the same time, move both arms leftward; the right palm travels downward and inward to the front of the abdomen, and the left palm travels inward so that it is level with the shoulders; the palms face each other. The eyes gaze horizontally at the right front.

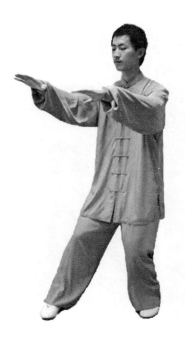
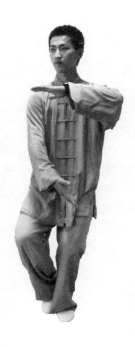

2. Continue rotating the waist rightward, step the right leg to the right front, touch the heel to the ground lightly, and shift the body weight forward slowly; plant the front foot solidly on the ground to form a right bow stance. At the same time, move the right palm forward and upward so that it is level with the forehead; the palm faces upward. Drop the left palm to the lower left, and press the palm down beside the left hip. The eyes gaze horizontally at the right palm.

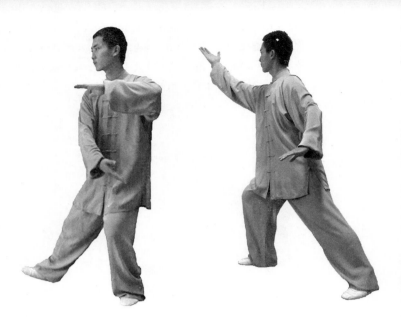

Movement 11: Fist Under the Elbow 肘底捶

1. Rotate the waist leftward while shifting the weight leftward, and pivot the right foot inward 120 degrees as the waist rotates. Rotate the waist rightward while shifting all the weight to the right foot, and draw the left foot back to the medial side of the right foot; touch the ball of the foot to the ground lightly. At the same time, move the right palm in front of the chest, passing the left shoulder; and move the left palm in front of the abdomen, passing the left hip. The palms face each other. The eyes gaze horizontally to the right front.

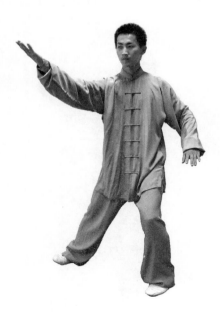

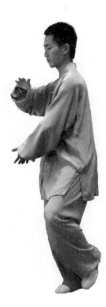

2. Rotate the waist leftward while stepping the left foot a half step to the left front; slowly shift the body weight to the left foot, then step the right foot forward a half step so that it is behind the left foot. At the same time, move both palms as the waist rotates; the left palm travels downward so that it is in front of the abdomen while the right palm goes upward so that it is in front of the forehead. The eyes gaze horizontally at the right hand.

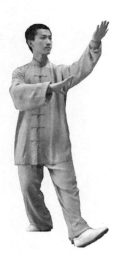 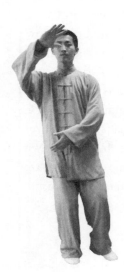

3. Rotate the waist rightward while shifting all the weight to the right leg; touch the left toes on the ground lightly. Rotate the left arm outward and raise it in front of the nose, while the right arm goes downward in front of the abdomen as it passes along the back of the left arm; turn the palms to face inward. Rotate the waist leftward as you lift the left toes, with the heel touching the ground lightly to form a left empty stance. At the same time, rotate the left palm inward as the waist rotates and lower it in the front of body so that it is chest-level; face the palm to the right. Simultaneously, change the right palm to a fist and draw it back under the left elbow, with the center of the fist facing left. The eyes gaze horizontally at the left hand.

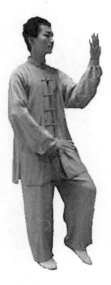 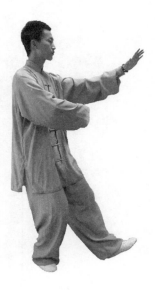

Movement 12: Step Back & Whirl Arms 倒卷肱

1. Rotate the waist rightward while changing the right fist to a palm; raise it backward and to the upper rear as it passes the waist, until the base of palm is ear-level; face the palm diagonally upward. As the waist rotates, the left arm rotates outward so that it is chest-level, with the palm facing upward. Eyes gaze horizontally at the right palm.

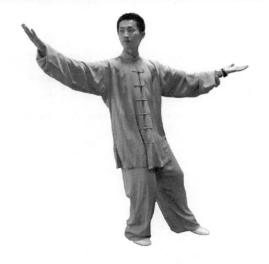

2. Rotate the waist leftward while shifting the body weight to the right foot; draw the left foot back to the medial side of the right foot. At the same time, draw the right palm inward beside the right ear; slightly withdraw the left palm downward. Eyes gaze at the left palm.

3. Continue to rotate the waist leftward. Step the left leg backward and shift the weight backward onto the left leg. At the same time, pivot on the ball of the foot so that the right toes point forward; the toes lightly contact the ground to form a right empty stance. As the waist rotates, push the right palm forward at chest-height with palm facing forward; bend the left elbow to withdraw the left arm so that it is in front of the abdomen, with palm facing upward. Eyes gaze horizontally at the right hand.

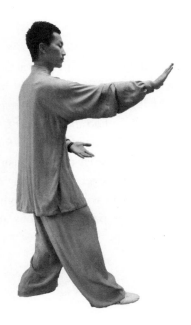

4. Rotate the waist leftward. Raise the left palm diagonally backward to the upper left rear so that it is ear-level; rotate both arms so that the palms face upward. The eyes gaze horizontally at the left palm.

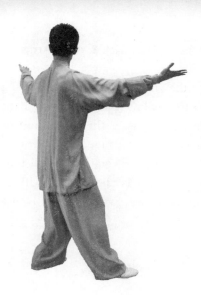

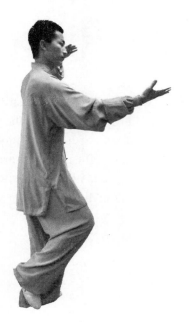

5. Rotate the waist rightward. Shift the body weight to the left foot, drawing the right foot back to the medial side of the left foot. At the same time, draw the left palm inward beside the left ear; withdraw the right palm downward slightly. Eyes gaze at the right palm.

6. Continue rotating the waist rightward. Step the right leg backward, shifting the weight backward onto the right leg. At the same time, pivot on the ball of the left foot so that the left toes point forward and touch the ground lightly to form a left empty stance. As the waist rotates, push the left palm forward at chest-level, palm facing forward; bend the right elbow to withdraw the right arm in front of the abdomen, palm facing upward. Eyes gaze horizontally at the left hand.

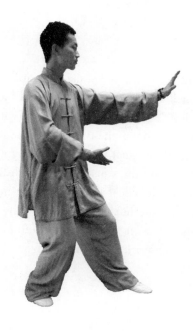

Movement 13: Work Shuttle (Left & Right) 左右穿梭

1. Rotate the waist rightward. At the same time, slightly shift the weight rightward, turning the left foot inward 120 degrees so that the toes point slightly toward each other. Slowly shift the weight to the left leg, and turn the right foot outward 120 degrees by pivoting on the heel; then, shift all the weight to the right foot, and draw the left foot back to the medial side of the right foot. Simultaneously, as the waist rotates, raise the right palm in front of the chest and drop the left palm in front of the abdomen; the palms face each other as if holding a ball. The eyes gaze horizontally at the left front.

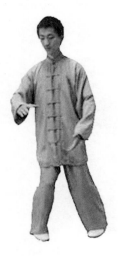
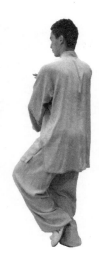

2. Step the left foot to the left front, touching the heel lightly on the ground. Slowly shift the weight forward, planting the front foot solidly on the ground to form a left bow stance. At the same time, while turning the waist leftward, rotate the left arm inward and raise it to the left front above the forehead, with the palm facing outward. Simultaneously, push the right palm to the left front, palm facing forward and fingers pointing upward. The eyes gaze horizontally at the right hand.

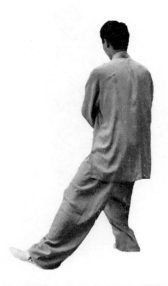
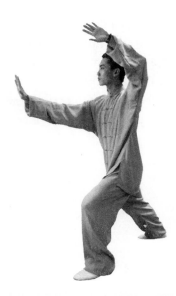

3. Rotate the waist leftward, turning the left foot outward 45 degrees, then shift all the weight to the left leg; draw the right foot back to the medial side of the right foot, with the toes lightly touching the ground. As the waist rotates, lower the right arm in front of the abdomen and lower the left arm in front of the chest; the palms face each other. The eyes gaze horizontally at the left front.

4. Step the right foot to the left front, with the heel lightly touching the ground. Slowly shift the body weight forward, planting the front foot solidly on the ground to form a right bow stance. At the same time, rotate the waist rightward, and rotate the right arm while raising it to the right front above the forehead, with palm facing outward. Simultaneously, push the left palm to the right front, with palm facing forward and fingers pointing upward. The eyes gaze horizontally at the left hand.

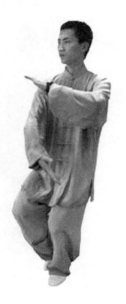

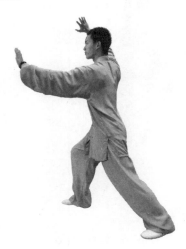

Movement 14: Part the Wild Horse's Mane (Left & Right) 左右野马分鬃

1. Rotate the waist rightward, turn the right foot outward 45 degrees, and slowly shift the weight to the right leg. Draw the left foot back to the medial side of the right foot, lightly touching the toes on the ground. At the same time, lower the left palm in front of the abdomen and the right arm in front of the chest; the palms face each other. The eyes gaze horizontally to the right front.

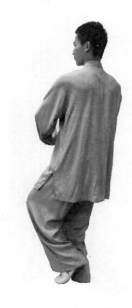

2. Step the left foot forward to the left, with the heel lightly contacting the ground. Slowly shift the body weight forward, and plant the front foot solidly on the ground to form a left bow stance. At the same time, rotate the waist leftward and raise the left arm to the left front until the base of the palm is chest-level; press the right palm downward beside the right hip. The eyes gaze horizontally at the left palm.

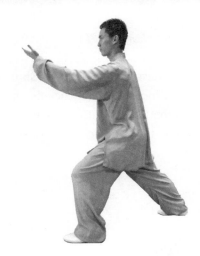

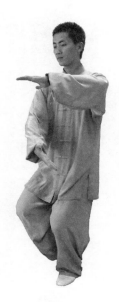

3. Rotate the waist leftward, turning the left foot outward 45 degrees, and shift the weight slowly to the left leg; then, draw the right foot to the medial side of the left foot, with toes lightly touching the ground. At the same time, move the right palm leftward in front of the abdomen and the left arm in front of the chest; the palms face each other. The eyes gaze horizontally to the left front.

4. Step the right foot forward to the right, touching the heel lightly on the ground. Slowly shift the body weight forward, planting the front foot solidly on the ground to form a right bow stance. At the same time, rotate the waist rightward, move the right arm to the right front until the base of palm is chest-level. Simultaneously, press the left palm downward beside the left hip. The eyes gaze horizontally at the right palm.

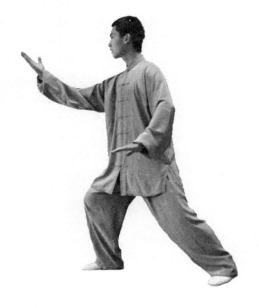

Movement 15: Wave Hands Like Clouds 云手

1. Rotate the waist leftward. Slowly shift the body weight to the left leg, and lift the right heel so that the ball of the foot lightly touches the ground. As the waist turns, rotate the left arm inward and raise it upward to the left side of the body until the base of palm is shoulder-level. At the same time, move the right arm to the left side of the waist as it passes the abdomen. The eyes gaze horizontally at the left palm.

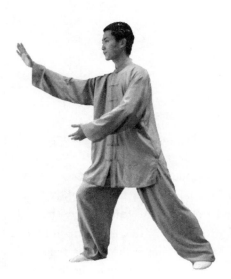
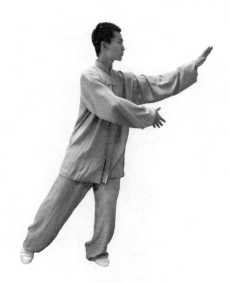

2. Rotate the waist rightward. Slowly shift the body weight to the right leg, and lift the left heel so that the ball of the foot contacts the ground lightly. As the waist turns, rotate the right arm inward and move it to the right side of the body as it passes the front of the body, and until the base of the palm is shoulder-level. At the same time, move the left arm to the right side of the waist as it passes the abdomen. Eyes gaze horizontally at the right palm.

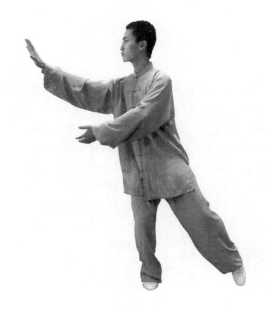

3. Same as step 1 in this movement.   4. Same as step 2 in this movement.   5. Same as step 1 in this movement.

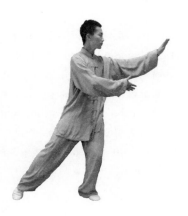 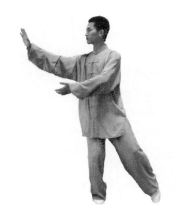 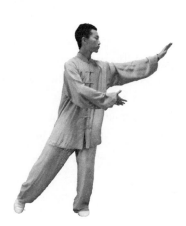

Movement 16: Single Whip   单鞭

Rotate the waist rightward. As the waist rotates, move the right arm to the right side as it passes the front of the body until the base of the palm is shoulder-level. At the same time, move the left palm to the medial side of the right arm as it passes the abdomen. Join the five fingers of the right hand together and bend the wrist to form a hook, with the wrist at ear-level. Rotate the waist leftward, shift all the body weight to the right leg, and move the left leg to the left front of the waist; touch the heel lightly on the ground. Slowly shift the body weight forward and plant the front foot solidly on the ground to form a left bow stance. At the same time, rotate the waist leftward and move the left palm in front of the left shoulder; push it forward with the base of the palm at shoulder-level. The eyes gaze horizontally at the left hand.

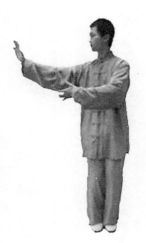 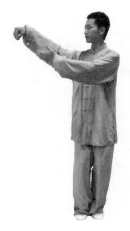 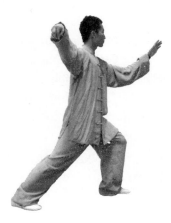

Movement 17: Pat High on Horse   高探马

1. Shift the body weight forward, step the right foot a half step forward so it is behind the left foot. At the same time, change the (right) hook into a palm. Rotate the waist rightward, and rotate both palms and arms outward as waist turns, with palm facing upward. The eyes gaze at the right palm.

2. Rotate the waist leftward, slowly shifting the body weight to the right leg and lift the left heel so that the ball of the foot touches the ground lightly to form a left empty stance. As the waist rotates, push the right palm forward as it passes the right ear. Simultaneously, draw the left palm slowly back in front of the abdomen. The eyes gaze horizontally at the right hand.

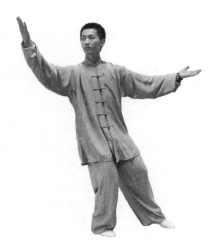
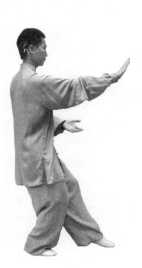

Movement 18: Right Heel Kick   右蹬脚

1. Rotate the waist leftward and draw the left foot back to the medial side of the right foot, then take a half step to the left front and shift the weight forward to form a left bow stance (while also rotating the waist rightward). Simultaneously, circle the palms in a clockwise direction 360 degrees and return them to the starting position. Eyes gaze horizontally at the right hand.

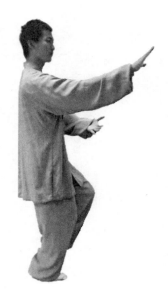
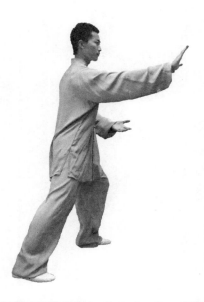

2. Rotate the waist leftward. Lower the right hand leftward in front of the chest and raise the left hand rightward in front of the chest so that the two cross at chest-level; the palms face inward, with the right palm outside the left palm. Simultaneously, raise the right knee. The eyes gaze at the left front.

3. Rotate the waist rightward. Kick the right leg to the right front, with force focused on the heel. Move the hands as the waist rotates, the left palm going to the left side of the body and the right palm to the right front, with both palms facing outward and the fingers pointing upward at shoulder-level. The eyes gaze horizontally at the right hand.

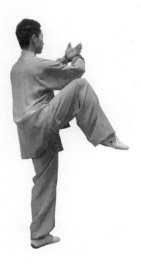

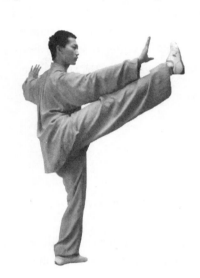

Movement 19: Double-strike the Ears   双风贯耳

1. Lift the right knee; at the same time, rotate the arms outward and move them horizontally in front of the body, arms level and shoulder-width apart, with fingers pointing forward. The eyes gaze horizontally at the palms.

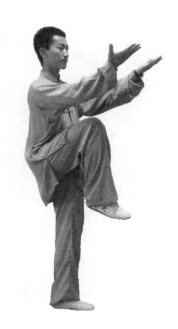

2. Lower the right leg on the ground to the right front, with the heel touching the ground lightly. At the same time, withdraw the palms beside the waist. Slowly shift the weight forward, planting the front foot solidly on the ground to form a right bow stance. Simultaneously, change the palms to fists as they circle outward, forward and then inward in front of the forehead. The eyes of the fists face each other, and the distance between the fists are slightly wider than the shoulders. The eyes gaze horizontally to the right front.

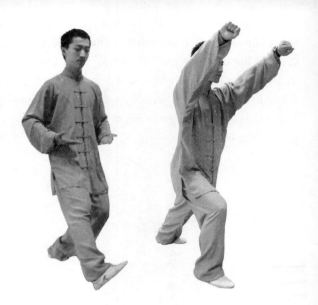

Movement 20: Left Toe Kick 左分脚

1. Rotate the waist rightward and sink the weight backward, while turning the right toes outward 45 degrees; at the same time, change the fists into palms, separate and move them diagonally upward to the side of the body. The palms face outward with the base of the palms at ear-level. Shift the body weight forward and draw the left foot to the medial side of the right foot, with toes touching the ground lightly. At the same time, rotate the waist rightward and lower the palms inward in front of the abdomen, with the right hand on the inside. The eyes gaze horizontally forward.

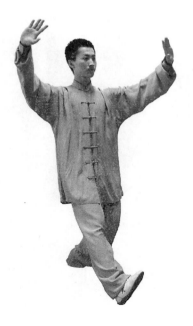
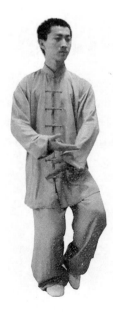

2. Lift the left knee. At the same time, cross the hands and raise them in front of the chest, with the left palm on the outside. Eyes gaze at the palms.

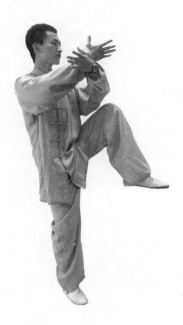

3. Rotate the waist leftward, and kick by straightening the left leg. At the same time, move the left palm forward to the left front and the right palm backward to the right rear, with both palms facing outward and the wrists at shoulder-level. Eyes gaze horizontally at the left hand.

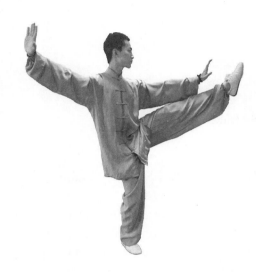

Movement 21: Turn Body & Heel Kick 转身蹬脚

1. Relax the left foot and lower it to the medial side of the right foot; at the same time, pivot on the ball of the right foot and turn the body around to the right using the momentum produced by the leg movement[14]. As the body turns, cross the palms in front of the abdomen as holding something, with right palm on the outside. Shift the weight to the left leg, and raise the arms to chest-level. The eyes gaze horizontally forward.

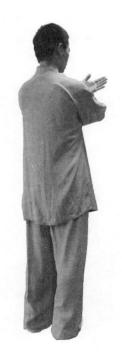

[14] The body turns clockwise 360 degrees in this movement.

2. Lift the right knee and kick
the right leg forward to the right
front, directing the force to the
heel. At the same time, rotate the
waist right, and move the arms
horizontally to the sides with
the left palm traveling to the left
side of body and the right palm
to the right front. The base of
the palms are shoulder-level,
with palms facing outward. The
eyes gaze horizontally at the
right hand.

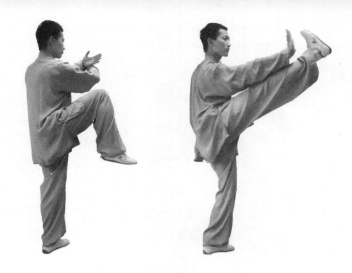

Movement 22: Needle at Sea Bottom 海底针

1. Rotate the waist rightward. Move the right foot
behind the left foot and plant it on the ground.
Shift the weight to the right leg, while the ball of
the left foot contacts the ground lightly to form a
left empty stance. As the waist rotates, draw the
right palm beside the right ear. The palm faces
left, with fingers pointing diagonally downward.
At the same time, press the left palm downward in
front of the abdomen, pointing the fingers toward
the right with palm facing downward. Eyes gaze
horizontally at the right palm.

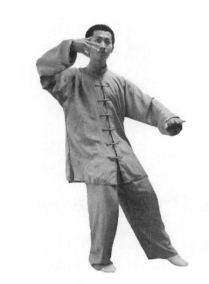

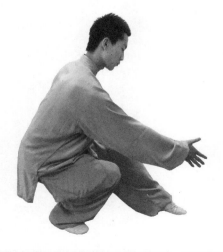

2. Rotate the waist leftward, and bend the knees to
squat, while extending the right arm downward to
the lower front as the waist rotates. Simultaneously,
press the left palm down beside the left knee. The
eyes gaze to right palm.

Movement 23: Deflect through the Back   闪通背

1. Rotate the waist rightward and raise the arms forward, pressing the four fingers of the left hand on the medial side of the right forearm; lift the left heel and touch the ball of the foot to the ground lightly.

2. Step the left foot forward, touching the heel on the ground lightly. Slowly shift the body weight forward, and plant the front foot solidly on the ground to form a left bow stance. At the same time, rotate the waist rightward while the right arm is raised to the right front above the forehead with the palm facing outward. Push the left hand forward with palm facing outward. The eyes gaze horizontally at the left hand.

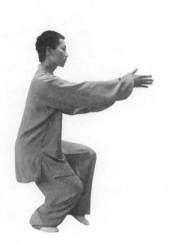 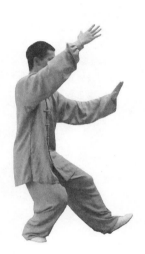 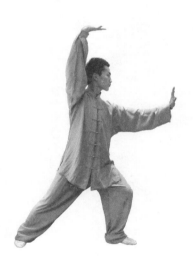

Movement 24: White Snake Spits Tongue   白蛇吐信

1. Shift the body weight to the right leg, and rotate the waist rightward. As the waist rotates, turn the left toes inward 120 degrees, then shift the weight to the left leg and draw the right foot back to the medial side of the left foot. Continue rotating the waist rightward. Change the right palm to a fist and move it inward in front of the abdomen with the eye of the fist facing downward; at the same time, raise the left palm above the forehead, with the palm facing outward. The eyes gaze horizontally to the right front.

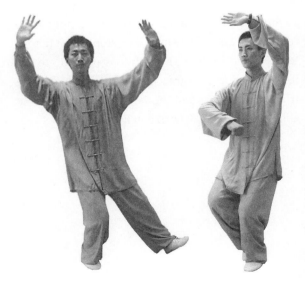

2. Continue rotating the waist rightward. Step the right foot to the right front, touching the heel lightly on the ground. Then, slowly shift the body weight forward, and plant the front foot solidly on the ground to form a right bow stance. At the same time, change the right fist to a palm and withdraw it downward to the right side of the waist as it passes the chest; point the fingers forward and face the palm upward. Push the left palm forward. The eyes gaze horizontally to the left palm.

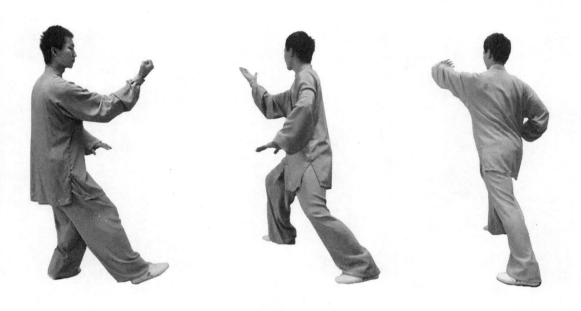

Movement 25: Right Slap Kick 右拍脚

1. Shift all the weight forward to the right foot, rotate the waist leftward, and step the left foot forward and to the right with toes pointing to the left. At the same time, move the right palm in front of the chest and the left arm in front of the abdomen; eyes gaze horizontally forward.

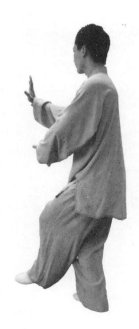

2. Continue shifting the weight forward until the entire weight of the body is loaded onto the left foot. Lift the right knee; at the same time, draw a 360-degree circle in a clockwise direction with both palms; then, cross the palms in front of the chest, with the right arm on the outside; face both palms inward; eyes gaze horizontally at the right front.

3. Flex the right instep so that the toes point forward, but in a relaxed manner, and kick toward the upper right front; at the same time, slap the right palm against the right instep; simultaneously, move the left palm backward to the rear left. The eyes gaze horizontally at the right hand.

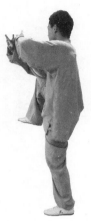

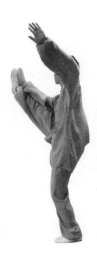

Movement 26: Subdue Tiger (Left & Right) 左右伏虎势

1. Step the right foot back to the medial side of the left foot, contacting the ground lightly. Then, sink the weight down on the right leg while drawing the right arm slightly inward at chest-level. At the same time, move the left palm forward to the medial side of the right elbow; bend both arms slightly with the palms facing downward. The eyes gaze horizontally at the right hand.

2. Rotate the waist leftward while shifting the weight to the right foot. Then, step the left foot forward to the left rear, with the heel touching the ground lightly. At the same time, move both arms to the left side of the body. Eyes gaze at the left palm.

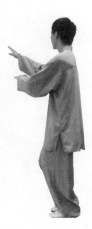

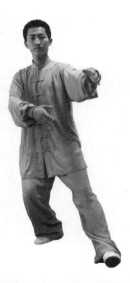

3. Continue rotating the waist leftward. Slowly shift the weight forward, planting the front foot solidly on the ground to form a left bow stance. At the same time, change both hands to fists, raising the left fist to the upper left above the forehead, with the eyes of the fist facing outward. Simultaneously, move the right fist leftward in front of the chest, with the center of the fist facing inward. Eyes gaze horizontally to the right front.

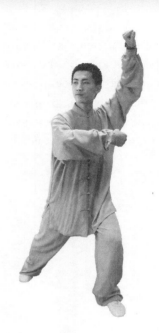

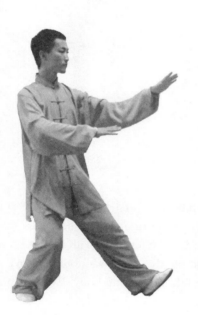

4. Shift the weight backward, rotating the waist rightward. At the same time, change the right fist to a palm and lower it slightly; change the left fist to a palm and lower it to shoulder-height; both palms face downward. Eyes gaze horizontally at the left hand.

5. Rotate the waist rightward and shift the body weight slowly to the left leg; step the right leg forward, touching the heel on the ground lightly. At the same time, move both arms to the right front.

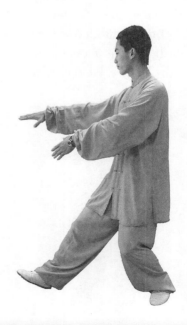

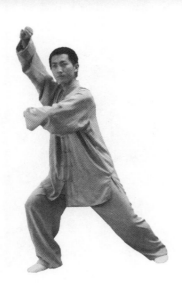

6. Continue rotating the waist rightward and slowly shift the weight forward, planting the front foot solidly on the ground to form a right bow stance. At the same time, change both hands to fists, raising the right fist to the upper right above the forehead, with the eye of the fist facing outward. Simultaneously, move the left fist rightward in front of the chest, with the center of the fist facing inward. Eyes gaze horizontally to the left front.

Movement 27: Crouch Down (Right) 右下势

1. Rotate the waist leftward while shifting the weight on the left leg as you turn the left toes outward 45 degrees. At the same time, change the left fist to a palm and move it backward to the rear left as it passes the abdomen. Then, bend the left wrist and change the palm to a hook, with the wrist at ear-level. Simultaneously, change the right fist to a palm and, as the waist turns, move it leftward in front of the left shoulder. Eyes gaze at the right hook.

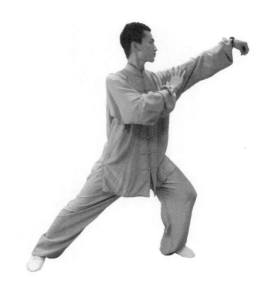

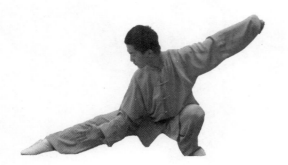

2. Bend the left knee to squat and straighten the right leg to form a right crouch stance. At the same time, extend the right palm forward, passing the chest, and move it along the medial side of the right leg. Eyes gaze at the right index finger.

金鸡独立

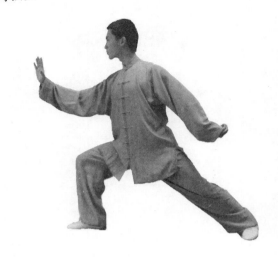

1. Shift the body weight forward, bend the right leg, and straighten the left leg to form a right bow stance. At the same time, continue extending the right palm forward. Simultaneously, rotate the left arm inward, with the tip of the left hook pointing upward. Eyes gaze horizontally at the right hand.

2. Shift the weight forward onto the right leg, and lift the left knee. At the same time, rotate the waist rightward, while pressing the right palm downward beside the right hip. Simultaneously, change the left hook to a palm, raising it forward and upward as if lifting something, while sinking the left elbow so that it is level with the left knee. The left palm and left knee should appear linked as they go up. The eyes gaze horizontally at the left palm.

3. Lower the left foot next to the medial side of the right foot; shift the weight to the left leg, and lift the right knee. At the same time, rotate the waist leftward and raise the right palm forward and upward as if lifting something, while sinking the right elbow so that it is level with the right knee. Simultaneously, press the left palm downward beside the left hip. Eyes gaze horizontally at the right palm.

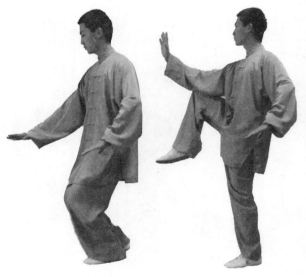

Movement 29: Bow Stance & Strike Groin 弓步指裆

1. Step the right foot forward, rotating the waist rightward while touching the heel on the ground; turn the toes outward as the waist rotates, then shift the weight forward onto the right leg. Draw the left foot to the medial side of the right foot, with the toes lightly touching the ground. At the same time, withdraw the right palm to the right side of the waist, and move the left palm forward with the base of the palm at chest-level. Step the left foot forward, with heel touching the ground lightly. The eyes gaze horizontally at the left hand.

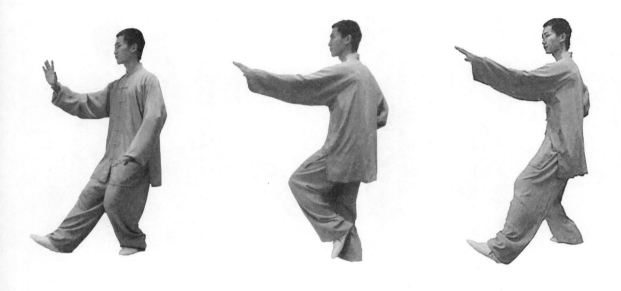

2. Rotate the waist leftward, shifting the body weight forward to form a left bow stance. As the waist turns, move the left arm slightly leftward to the outside of the left knee. Simultaneously, change the right palm to a fist and punch forward and downward, with the eye of the fist facing upward. The eyes gaze at the right fist.

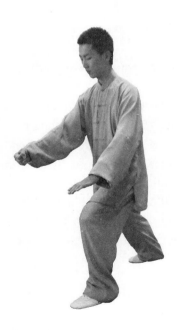

> Movement 30: Grasp the Sparrow's Tail   揽雀尾

Rotate the waist leftward while turning the left foot outward 45 degrees, and shift the body weight forward onto the left leg. While the waist rotates, change the right fist to a palm, and move both arms to the left in front of the abdomen. Then, raise the arms so that they cross in front of the chest, with the right arm on the outside. Eyes gaze horizontally forward.

The remaining specifications and key points are the same as in "Movement 2b: Grasp the Sparrow's Tail."

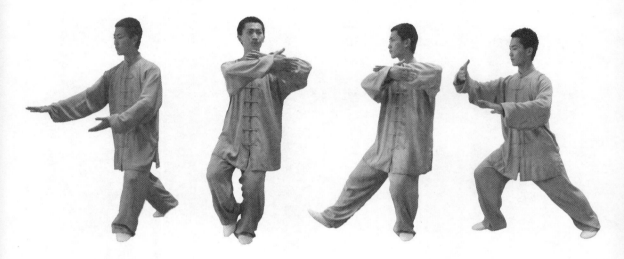

> Movement 31: Single Whip   单鞭

The specifications and key points for movements are the same as in the previous "Single Whip" (Movement 3).

> Movement 32: Crouch Down (Left)   左下势

Rotate the waist rightward while turning the right toes outward 45 degrees, and align the right knee outward at the same angle. Then, bend the right knee and squat, while straightening the left leg to form a left crouch stance. At the same time, draw the left palm upward and inward in front of the left side of the chest, then extend it forward, passing the chest and along the medial side of the left leg. The eyes gaze at the left palm.

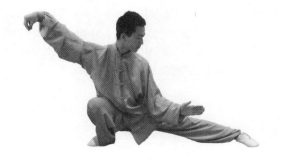

Movement 33: Step Forward to Seven Stars 上步七星

Turn the left toes outward 90 degrees, and slowly stand up and straighten the body; then, slowly shift the weight forward to the left leg. At the same time, rotate the waist rightward, lift the right foot, and take a half step forward in front of the left foot, with toes lightly touching the ground, to form a right empty stance. Simultaneously, lower the right hook downward then forward, passing the chest and right hip, with the eye of the fist facing forward; at the same time, rotate the left palm outward and change it to a fist, with the center of the fist facing inward. Cross the fists in front of the chest, right fist on the outside; eyes gaze horizontally forward.

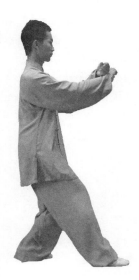

Movement 34: Step Back & Straddle the Tiger 退步跨虎

Rotate the waist rightward and step the right foot back to the right side behind the left foot. Shift the weight to the right leg, with the ball of the left foot lightly contacting the ground, to form a left empty stance. At the same time, change both fists to palms and lower them in front of the abdomen; then, separate them, with the right palm moving upward to the upper right above the forehead; the palm faces outward. Rotate the waist leftward to face forward and move the left palm downward to press beside the left hip. The eyes gaze horizontally forward.

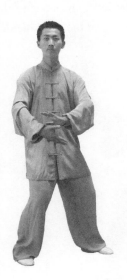
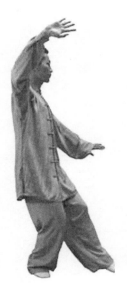
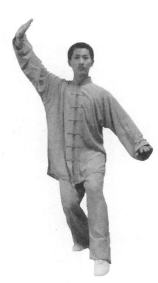

front view

Movement 35: Turn Body & Lotus Kick   转身摆莲

1. Rotate the waist rightward and point the left foot inward 120 degrees. At the same time, lower the right arm downward to the right side of the waist, and move the left palm forward in front of the body so that it is level with the shoulders. Eyes gaze at the left palm.

2. Continue rotating the waist rightward and shift the weight to the left leg. Step the right leg forward to the right rear; touch the heel on the ground, and turn the toes outward. At the same time, swing the right arm with the palm facing up and extend it to the right so that it is above the left arm. Simultaneously, swing the left arm to the right side of the body as the waist turns; eyes gaze to the right palm.

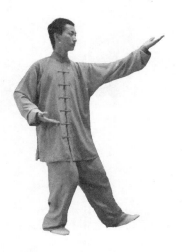

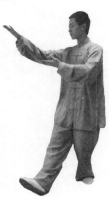

3. Continue rotating the waist rightward, shift the body weight to the right foot, and lower the left leg to the right front, with toes pointing inward as the left foot steps onto the ground. Then, shift the weight to the left leg, and step the right leg a half step forward, touching the toes on the ground lightly to form a right empty stance. At the same time, move the arms horizontally around the body, with the right palm to the right side of the body; the base of the palm is level with the shoulders; the left palm goes to the medial side of the right forearm, with palm facing inward. The eyes gaze horizontally at the right hand.

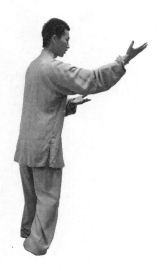

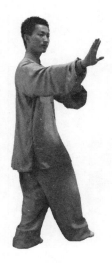

4. Slightly rotate the waist rightward, lift the right knee, then straighten the right leg and extend it to the upper right with the instep relaxed. At the same time, swing both palms from right to left to slap the right instep as the right leg swings from left to right.

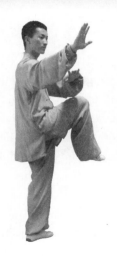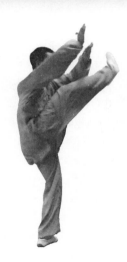

Movement 36: Bend Bow to Shoot Tiger 弯弓射虎

Lower and step the right foot down to the right, then rotate the waist rightward and shift the weight onto the right leg to form a right bow stance. At the same time, lower the palms to the right rear. Next, rotate the waist leftward, and change the palms to fists as they move to the left following the rotation of the waist. Then, raise the right fist to the upper right above the forehead, with the eye of the fist facing outward; at the same time, punch the left fist to the left front, with center of fist facing downward. The eyes gaze at the right fist.

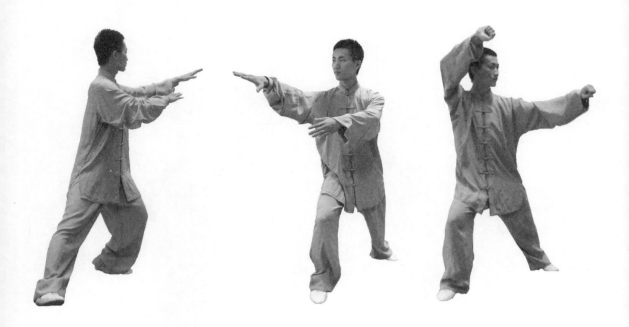

Movement 37: Parry & Punch 搬拦捶

Rotate the waist leftward, shift the body weight slightly to the right and turn the left foot outward 45 degrees; as the waist rotates, change the left fist to a palm and move it to front of the chest. At the same time, lower the right fist in front of the abdomen; shift the weight to the left leg, and step the right leg to the right front, with the heel lightly touching the ground. Then, rotate the waist rightward and turn the right toes outward 45 degrees; move the left palm rightward as the waist rotates. The left palm protects the medial side of the right elbow as the right fist punches forward; the left foot plants solidly on the ground. The eyes gaze horizontally at the right fist.

The remaining specifications and key points are the same as in "Movement 8: Parry and Punch."

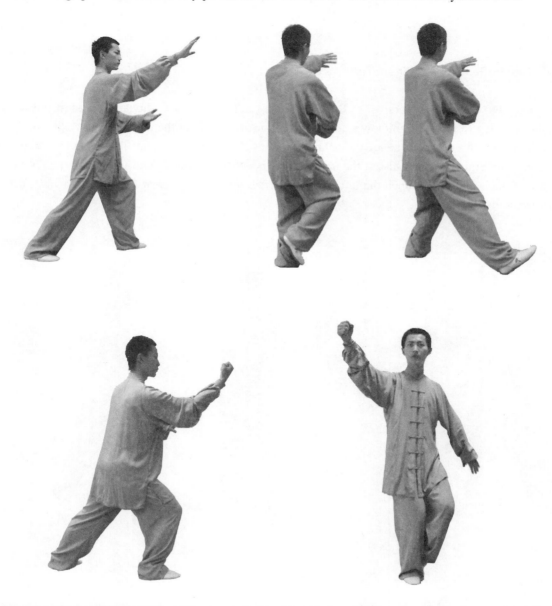

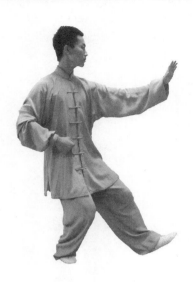
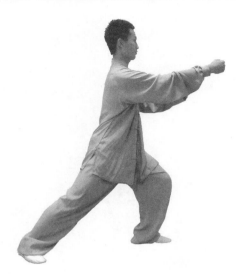

Movement 38: Apparent Close 如封四闭

The specification and keys of movements are the same as in "Movement 9: Apparent Close".

Movement 39: Cross Hands 十字手

1. Rotate the waist rightward while shifting the body weight to the right leg. Lift the left toes and turn them in the direction used in the opening movement. At the same time, bend the right knee, and move the right hand to the right horizontally so that the arms are on either side of the body; eyes gaze at the right palm.

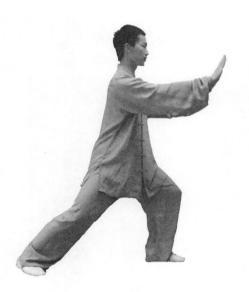
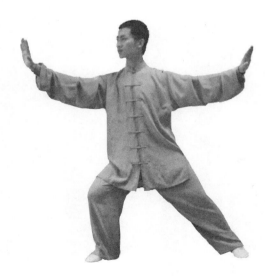

2. Rotate the waist leftward, shift all the weight to the left leg and draw the right foot back to the left a half step; at the same time, lower the hands inward to cross in front of the chest, with the left hand on top and the right hand on the outside. The eyes gaze at the palms.

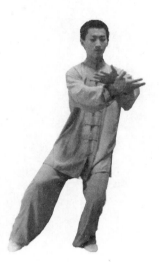 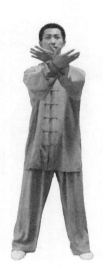

Movement 40: Closing   收势

Rotate the arms inward so that the palms face downward, and extend them forward. Lower the hands to the sides of the thighs. Shift all the weight to the right leg, draw the left foot to the medial side of the right foot, then plant it on the ground. Distribute the weight evenly between both legs, relax the arms and let them hang loosely alongside the body. Eyes gaze forward.

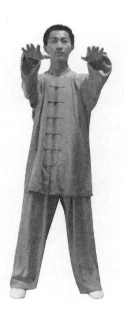 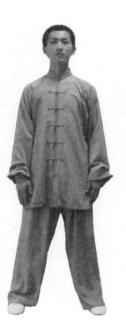 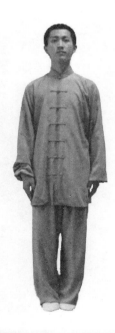

Chapter 8
Common Mistakes in Tai Ji Quan Practice

1. Feet Not Parallel

Detail: Toes pointing outward so they form the Chinese character for eight (八).

To correct the mistake: Point the toes forward, and stand with the feet parallel.

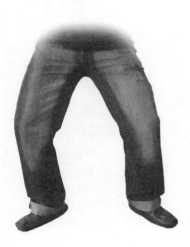 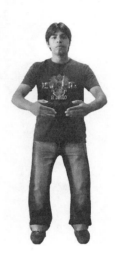

2. Knees Overly Bent

Detail: Knees are bent too much so they protrude beyond the tips of the toes.

To correct the mistake: Relax the waist and retract the buttocks; shift the body weight backward and downward, so that the knee joints do not go beyond the tips of the toes.

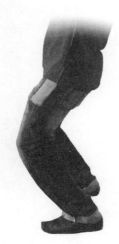 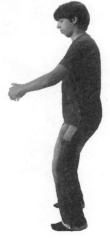

3. Waist Bent

Detail: The spine and tailbone are not straight; and the body leans forward or backward.

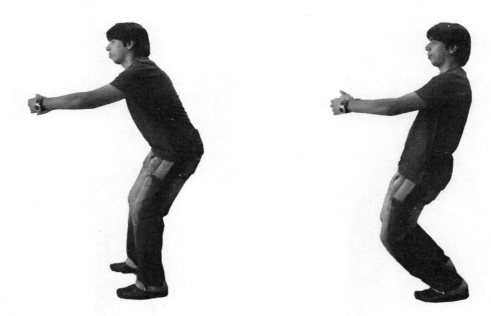

To correct the mistake: Relax the waist and the area along the spine at DU 4 (*mìng mén*, 命门); retract the hips and buttocks, and straighten the upper body.

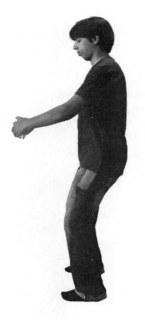
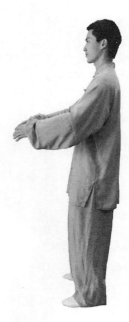

4. Shoulders Shrugged and Elbows Raised

Detail: The shoulders are tense and the elbow joints are raised.

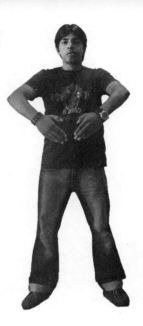

To correct the mistake: Sink the qi to the elixir field (*dān tián*); sink the shoulders and drop the elbows so that the upper limbs form a smooth circular arc.

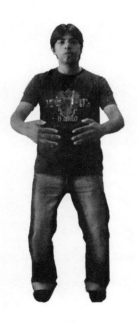

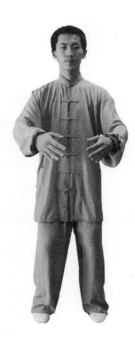

5. Head is Dropped or Raised

Detail: The neck (cervical vertebrae) bends forward or backward and is not perpendicular to the ground.

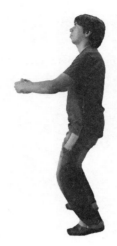
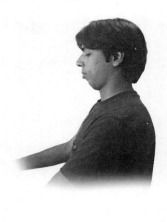

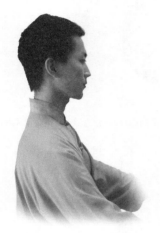

To correct the mistake: Draw the chin slightly toward the neck, push the vertex of the head at DU 20 (*bǎi huì*, 百会) upward, and straighten the neck; look horizontally forward, and relax the shoulders.

6. Underarms are Constricted

Detail: The upper arms stick to the body.
To correct the mistake: Relax the area under the arms; keep the upper arms one fist's distance from the body.

7. Body is Unsteady when Shifting Weight

Detail: Body is unsteady when shifting body weight.
To correct the mistake: Relax the body and limbs, and shift the body weight at a slow pace to reduce obvious up and down movements.

8. Body Leans while Shifting Weight

Detail: Body leans backward while shifting the body weight backward, and leans forward while shifting the weight forward.
To correct the mistake: Relax the waist and keep the body upright; move the body on a horizontal plane while shifting weight.

Appendix:
Yang Style Tai Ji Quan Routines

1. The 8 Movements Routine 八式太极拳拳谱

1. Whirl Arms　　　　　　　　　　卷肱势
2. Twist Step & Brush Knee　　　　搂膝拗步
3. Part The Wild Horse's Mane　　　野马分鬃
4. Wave Hands Like Clouds　　　　云手
5. Golden Cock Stands On One Leg　金鸡独立
6. Heel Kick　　　　　　　　　　蹬脚
7. Grasp The Sparrow's Tail　　　　揽雀尾
8. Cross Hands　　　　　　　　　十字手

2. The 16 Movements Routine 十六式太极拳拳谱

1. Opening　　　　　　　　　　　起势
2. Part the Wild Horse's Mane (Left & Right)　左右野马分鬃
3. White Crane Spreads Wings　　　白鹤亮翅
4. Twist Step & Brush Knee (Left & Right)　左右搂膝拗步
5. Step Forward & Parry and Punch　进步搬拦捶
6. Apparent Close　　　　　　　　如封似闭
7. Single Whip　　　　　　　　　单鞭
8. Hands Strum the Lute　　　　　手挥琵琶
9. Step Back & Whirl Arms　　　　倒卷肱
10. Work Shuttle (Left & Right)　　左右穿梭
11. Needle at Sea Bottom　　　　　海底针
12. Deflect through the Back　　　　闪通背
13. Wave Hands Like Clouds　　　　云手
14. Grasp the Sparrow's Tail (Left & Right)　左右揽雀尾
15. Cross Hands　　　　　　　　　十字手
16. Closing　　　　　　　　　　　收势

3. The 24 Movements Routine 二十四式太极拳拳谱

1. Opening　　　　　　　　　　　起式
2. Part the Wild Horse's Mane (Left & Right)　左右野马分鬃
3. White Crane Spreads Wings　　　白鹤亮翅
4. Twist Step & Brush Knee (Left & Right)　左右搂膝拗步
5. Hands Strum the Lute　　　　　手挥琵琶

6. Step Back & Whirl Arms (Left & Right)   左右倒卷肱
7. Grasp The Sparrow's Tail (Left)   左揽雀尾
8. Grasp The Sparrow's Tail (Right)   右揽雀尾
9. Single Whip   单鞭
10. Wave Hands Like Clouds   云手
11. Single Whip   单鞭
12. Pat High on Horse   高探马
13. Right Heel Kick   右蹬脚
14. Double-strike the Ears   双峰贯
15. Turn Body & Left Heel Kick   转身左蹬脚
16. Crouch Down (Left) & Stand on One Leg   左下势独立
17. Crouch Down (Right) & Stand on One Leg   右下势独立
18. Work Shuttle (Left & Right)   左右穿梭
19. Needle at Sea Bottom   海底针
20. Deflect Through the Back   闪通背
21. Turn Body, Parry & Punch   转身搬拦捶
22. Apparent Close   如封似闭
23. Cross Hands   十字手
24. Closing   收势

4. The 32 Movements Routine   三十二式太极拳拳谱

Ready Posture   预备式
1. Opening   起势
2. Grasp the Sparrow's Tail Right   右揽雀尾
3. Left Single Whip   左单鞭
4. Hands Strum the Lute   琵琶势
5. Step Forward & Parry and Punch   进步搬拦捶
6. Apparent Close   如封似闭
7. Twist Step & Brush Knee   搂膝拗步
8. Single Whip Right   右单鞭
9. Wave Hands Like Clouds Right   右云手
10. Part the Wild Horse's Mane   野马分鬃
11. Needle at Sea Bottom   海底针
12. Deflect through the Back   闪通背
13. Grasp the Sparrow's Tail Right   右揽雀尾
14. Turn Body, Deflect & Punch   转体撇身捶
15. Roll Back & Press   捋挤势
16. Right Slap Kick   右拍脚
17. Left Instep Kick   左分脚
18. Right Heel Kick   右蹬脚
19. Step Forward & Strike   进步栽捶
20. Work Shuttle on Left & Right   左右穿梭
21. Fist Under the Elbow   肘底捶

22. Step Back & Whirl Arms	倒卷肱
23. Crouch Down (Right)	右下势
24. Golden Cock Stands on One Leg	金鸡独立
25. Crouch Down (Left)	左下势
26. Step Forward to Seven Stars	上步七星
27. Step Back & Straddle the Tiger	退步跨虎
28. Turn Body & Lotus Kick	转身摆莲
29. Bend Bow to Shoot Tiger	弯弓射虎
30. Grasp the Sparrow's Tail (Left)	左揽雀尾
31. Cross Hands	十字手
32. Closing	收势

5. The 48 Movements Routine 四十八式太极拳拳谱

Ready Position	起势
1. White Crane Spreads Wings	白鹤亮翅
2. Twist Step & Brush Knee (Left)	左搂膝拗步
3. Single Whip (Left)	左单鞭
4. Hands Strum the Lute (Left)	左琵琶
5. Roll Back & Press	捋挤势
6. Deflect, Parry & Punch (Left)	左搬拦捶
7. Ward-Off, Roll Back, & Press & Push (Left)	左掤捋挤按
8. Diagonal Bump	斜身靠
9. Fist Under the Elbow	肘底捶
10. Step Back & Whirl Arms	倒卷肱
11. Turn Body & Push Palms	转身推掌
12. Hands Strum the Lute Right	右琵琶势
13. Brush Knee & Punch Down	搂膝栽捶
14. White Snake Spits Tongue	白蛇吐信
15. Slap Foot & Subdue Tiger	拍脚伏虎
16. Left Diagonal Back-fist	左撇身捶
17. Piercing Fist & Crouch Down	穿拳下势
18. Stand on One Leg & Prop-Up Palm	独立撑掌
19. Single Whip (Right)	右单鞭
20. Wave Hands Like Clouds (Right)	右云手
21. Part the Mane (Right & Left)	右左分鬃
22. Pat High on Horse	高探马
23. Right Heel Kick	右蹬脚
24. Double-strike the Ears	双峰贯耳
25. Left Heel Kick	左蹬脚
26. Guard Hands & Strike with Fist	掩手撩拳
27. Needle at Sea Bottom	海底针
28. Deflect through the Back	闪通背
29. Separate Legs (Right & Left)	右左分脚

30. Twist Step & Brush Knee   搂膝拗步
31. Step Forward, Catch & Strike   上步擒打
32. Apparent Close   如封似闭
33. Wave Hands Like Clouds (Left)   左云手
34. Right Diagonal Back-fist   右撇身捶
35. Work Shuttle on Left & Right   左右穿梭
36. Step Back & Spear Palm   退步穿掌
37. Empty Stance & Press Palms Down 虚步压掌
38. Stand on One Leg Raising Palm Up 独立托掌
39. Horse Stance & Bump   马步靠
40. Turn Body & Large Roll Back   转身大捋
41. Scoop Palm & Crouch Down   撩掌下势
42. Step Forward to Seven Stars   上步七星
43. Stand on One Leg & Straddle the Tiger 独立跨虎
44. Turn Body & Lotus Kick   转身摆莲
45. Bend Bow & Shoot Tiger   弯弓射虎
46. Right Parry & Punch   右搬拦捶
47. Ward-Off , Roll Back, Press & Push (Right) 右掤捋挤按
48. Cross Hands   十字手
     Closing & Return to Opening Posture 收势还原

6. The 88 Movements Routine   杨式88式太极拳拳谱

1. Ready Posture   预备式
2. Opening   起势
3. Grasp The Sparrow's Tail   揽雀尾
4. Single Whip   单鞭
5. Raise Hands   提手
6. White Crane Spreads Wings   白鹤亮翅
7. Twist Step & Brush Knee (Left)   左搂膝拗步
8. Hands Strum the Lute   手挥琵琶
9. Twist Step & Brush Knee (Left & Right) 左右搂膝拗步
10. Hands Strum the Lute   手挥琵琶
11. Step Forward, Deflect, Parry and Punch 进步搬拦捶
12. Apparent Close   如封似闭
13. Cross Hands   十字手
14. Embrace Tiger & Return to Mountain 抱虎归山
15. Grasp the Sparrow's Tail (Diagonal) 斜揽雀尾
16. Fist Under the Elbow   肘底看捶
17. Step Back & Whirl Arms (Left & Right) 左右倒卷肱
18. Diagonal Flying   斜飞式
19. Raise Hands   提手
20. White Crane Spreads Wings   白鹤亮翅
21. Twist Step & Brush Knee Left   左搂膝拗步

22. Needle at Sea Bottom   海底针
23. Deflect Through the Back   闪通背
24. Turn Body, Back-fist & Punch   转身撇身捶
25. Step Forward, Deflect, Parry and Punch   进步搬拦捶
26. Step Forward & Grasp the Sparrow's Tail   上步揽雀尾
27. Single Whip   单鞭
28. Wave Hands Like Clouds   云手
29. Single Whip   单鞭
30. Pat High on Horse   高探马
31. Separate & Kick Right   右分腿
32. Separate & Kick Left   左分腿
33. Turn Body & Left Heel Kick   转身左蹬腿
34. Twist Step & Brush Knee Left & Right   左右搂膝拗步
35. Step Forward & Punch Down   进步栽捶
36. Turn Body & White Snake Spits Tongue   翻身白蛇吐信
37. Step Forward & Deflect, Parry and Punch   进步搬拦捶
38. Right Heel Kick   右蹬腿
39. Subdue Tiger (Left)   左披身伏虎
40. Subdue Tiger (Right)   右披身伏虎
41. Turn Body & Right Heel Kick   回身右蹬腿
42. Double-strike the Ears   双峰贯耳
43. Left Heel Kick   左蹬腿
44. Turn Body & Right Heel Kick   转身右蹬腿
45. Step Forward, Deflect, Parry and Punch   进步搬拦捶
46. Apparent Close   如封似闭
47. Cross Hands   十字手
48. Embrace Tiger & Return to Mountain   抱虎归山
49. Grasp the Sparrow's Tail (Diagonal)   斜揽雀尾
50. Single Whip (Diagonal)   横单鞭
51. Part The Wild Horse's Mane (Left & Right)   左右野马分鬃
52. Step Forward & Grasp the Sparrow's Tail   进步揽雀尾
53. Single Whip   单鞭
54. Work Shuttle (Left & Right)   左右穿梭
55. Step Forward & Grasp the Sparrow's Tail   进步揽雀尾
56. Single Whip   单鞭
57. Wave Hands Like Clouds   云手
58. Single Whip   单鞭
59. Crouch Down   下势
60. Golden Cock Stands on One Leg (Left & Right) 左右金鸡独立
61. Step Back & Whirl Arms (Left & Right)   左右倒卷肱
62. Diagonal Flying   斜飞式
63. Raise Hands   提手
64. White Crane Spreads Wings   白鹤亮翅

65. Twist Step & Brush Knee (Left) 左搂膝拗步
66. Needle at Sea Bottom 海底针
67. Deflect Through the Back 闪通背
68. Turn Body, Back-fist & Punch 转身撇身捶
69. Step Forward, Deflect, Parry and Punch 进步搬拦捶
70. Step Forward & Grasp the Sparrow's Tail 上步揽雀尾
71. Single Whip 单鞭
72. Wave Hands Like Clouds 云手
73. Single Whip 单鞭
74. Pat High on Horse 高探马
75. Left Spear Palm 左穿掌
76. Turn Body, Cross Hands & Heel Kick 转身十字蹬腿
77. Brush Knee & Punch Down 搂膝打捶
78. Step Forward & Grasp the Sparrow's Tail 上步揽雀尾
79. Single Whip 单鞭
80. Crouch Down 下势
81. Step Forward to Seven Stars 上步七星
82. Step Back & Straddle the Tiger 退步跨虎
83. Turn Body & Lotus Kick 转身摆莲腿
84. Bend Bow & Shoot Tiger 弯弓射虎
85. Step Forward, Deflect, Parry and Punch 进步搬拦捶
86. Apparent Close 如封似闭
87. Cross Hands 十字手
88. Closing & Return to Opening Posture 收势还原

7. The Yang Style Old Frame Dynamic 128 Movements Routine
杨式老架动功太极拳128式拳谱

Part 1

1. Opening 起势
2. Lion Plays Ball 狮子滚球
3. Split & Collapse Mount Hua 分崩华山
4. White Snake Spits Tongue 白蛇吐信
5. Gentle Breeze Caresses the Willow 和风戏柳
6. Step Forward & Grasp the Sparrow's Tail 进步揽雀尾
7. Brush Knee (Right) 右搂膝
8. Palm Strikes Groin 沙掌击裆
9. Deflect through the Back 闪通背
10. Fish with Eagle Claw 鹰爪钓鱼
11. Single Whip 单鞭
12. Raise Hands & Step Forward 提手上式
13. White Crane Spreads Wings 白鹤亮翅
14. Snake Winds Around the Knee 蛇盘缠膝
15. Brush Knee (Right) 右搂膝

16. Hands Strum the Lute   手抱琵琶
17. Continuously Spear Palms   连环穿掌
18. Dragon Steps   龙行步
19. Step Forward, Deflect, Parry and Punch   进步搬拦捶
20. Golden Boy Worships Buddha   金童参佛

Part 2

21. Continuously Spear Palms   连环穿掌
22. Embrace Tiger & Return to Mountain   抱虎归山
23. Grasp the Sparrow's Tail   揽雀尾
24. Diagonal Single Whip   斜单鞭
25. Gentle Breeze Caresses the Willow   和风戏柳
26. Fist Under the Elbow   肘底看捶
27. Step Back & Whirl Arms   倒卷肱
28. Open Window to Look at the Moon   推窗望月
29. Fierce Tiger Returns to Cave   猛虎归洞
30. Diagonal Flying   斜飞式
31. Raise Hands & Step Up   提手上式
32. White Crane Spreads Wings   白鹤亮翅
33. Brush Knee (Left)   左搂膝
34. Scoop Moon from Sea Bottom   海底捞月
35. Agile Ape Guards the Cave   灵猿守洞
36. Palm Strikes Groin   沙掌击裆
37. Deflect through the Back   闪通背
38. Turn Over to Support Heaven and Earth   翻身顶天立地
39. Step Forward & Double-strike the Ears   上步双峰贯耳
40. Roc Spreads Wings   大鹏展翅
41. Step Forward & Grasp the Sparrow's Tail   上步揽雀尾
42. Single Whip   单鞭
43. Burst through the Black Clouds   拨开乌云
44. Palm Strikes Groin   沙掌击裆
45. Deflect through the Back   闪通背
46. Sparrow Hawk Turns Over   鹞子翻身
47. Split & Collapse Hua Mountain   分崩华山
48. Palm Strikes Groin   沙掌击裆
49. Deflect Through the Back   闪通背
50. Sparrow Hawk Turns Over   鹞子翻身
51. Split & Collapse Mount Hua   分崩华山
52. Pat High on Horse   高探马
53. Right Pierce-the-Heart Kick   右穿心脚
54. White Snake Spits Tongue   白蛇吐信
55. Left Pierce-the-Heart Kick   左穿心脚
56. Turn Body & Left Heel Kick   转身左蹬

57. Brush Knee (Left)   左搂膝
58. Brush Knee (Right)   右搂膝
59. Immortal Plays with Cicada   刘海戏蝉
60. Turn Over & Back-fist   翻身披身拳
61. Step Forward, Deflect Parry and Punch   进步搬拦捶
62. Right Heel Kick   右蹬脚
63. Palm Strike Groin   沙掌击裆
64. Hit Tiger (Palm) Middle   中打虎（掌）
65. Hit Tiger (Left)   左打虎
66. Hit Tiger (Fist) Middle   中打虎（拳）
67. Hit Tiger (Right)   右打虎
68. Right Heel Kick   右蹬脚
69. Two Dragons Fight for Pearl   双龙夺珠
70. Left Heel Kick   左蹬脚
71. Tornado & Lotus Kick   旋风摆莲
72. Gentle Breeze Caresses the Willow   和风戏柳
73. Right Heel Kick   右蹬脚
74. Dragon Boat Tours Palace   龙船游宫
75. Part the Wild Horse's Mane   野马分鬃
76. Step Forward & Parry and Punch   进步搬拦捶
77. Golden Boy Worships Buddha   金童参佛

Part 3

78. Continuously Spear Palm   连环穿掌
79. Embrace Tiger & Return to Mountain   抱虎归山
80. Grasp the Sparrow's Tail   揽雀尾
81. Diagonal Single Whip   斜单鞭
82. Part the Wild Horse's Mane   野马分鬃
83. Step Forward & Grasp the Sparrow's Tail   上步揽雀尾
84. Diagonal Single Whip   斜单鞭
85. Part the Wild Horse's Mane   野马分鬃
86. Jade Girl Works Shuttle   玉女穿梭
87. Step Forward & Grasp the Sparrow's Tail   上步揽雀尾
88. Split & Collapse Mount Hua   分崩华山
89. Sleeping Dragon Crouches Down   卧龙下势
90. Blue Dragon Flies   青龙飞腾
91. Phoenix Comes out from Nest   凤凰出巢
92. Golden Cock Stands on One Leg   金鸡独立
93. Step Back & Whirl Arms   倒卷肱
94. Open Window to Look at the Moon   推窗望月
95. Fierce Tiger Returns to Cave   猛虎归洞
96. Diagonal Flying   斜飞式
97. Raise Hands & Step Up   提手上式

98. White Crane Spreads Wings   白鹤亮翅
99. Twist Step & Brush Knee (Left)   左搂膝拗步
100. Scoop the Moon from Sea Bottom   海底捞月
101. Agile Ape Guards Cave   灵猿守洞
102. Palm Strikes Groin   沙掌击裆
103. Deflect Through the Back   闪通背
104. Turn & Back-fist   翻身披身拳
105. Deflect, Parry & Punch   搬拦拳
106. Horse Stance Creates Power   马步行功
107. Step Forward & Grasp the Sparrow's Tail   上步揽雀尾
108. Single Whip   单鞭
109. Wave Hands Like Clouds & Whirlwind   云手旋轮
110. Single Whip   单鞭
111. Pat High on Horse & Spear Hand   高探马穿掌
112. Turn Body & Right Heel Kick   翻身右蹬脚
113. Step Forward & Punch Groin   进步指裆捶
114. Horse Stance Creates Power   马步行功
115. Step Forward & Grasp the Sparrow's Tail   上步揽雀尾
116. Split & Collapse Mount Hua   分崩华山
117. Sleeping Dragon Crouches Down   卧龙下势
118. Seven Stars & Hang the Lantern   七星挂灯
119. Step Back & Straddle the Tiger   退步跨虎
120. Open Window to Look at the Moon   推窗望月
121. Fierce Tiger Return to Cave   猛虎归洞
122. Rotate Body & Double Lotus Kick   旋身双摆莲
123. Bend Bow & Shoot Tiger   弯弓射虎
124. Hunt Tiger (Left)   左打虎势
125. Step Forward and Deflect, Parry and Punch   进步搬拦拳
126. Golden Boy Worships Buddha   金童参佛
127. Reverse Yin and Yang   反转阴阳
128. Closing Tai Ji Posture   合太极式

References

1. Chen Qing-shan, Hu Lai-dong. The Influence of Taoist Philosophy on Tai Ji Quan Theories (道家哲学思想对太极拳理论的影响). *Journal of Adult Sports Education*. 2004 (02).

2. Chen Xin. *Illustrated Chen Style Tai Ji Quan* (陈氏太极拳图说). Shanxi: Shanxi Science and Technology Press; 2006.

3. Feng Ling, Feng Yun-xia, Xing Xiao-hu. Tai Ji Quan is the Best Dynamic Practice to Cultivate Both Body and Personality (太极拳是性命双修的最好动功). *Chinese Martial Arts*. 2004 (02).

4. Guo Zhi-yu. A Study of the Tai Ji Quan Health Cultivation Culture (太极拳养生文化考). *Journal of Shanghai Sports Institute*. 2004 (02).

5. Wei Shu-ren. *The Core Teachings of Tai Ji Quan* (太极拳行拳心法). Beijing: People's Sports Publishing House; 2001.

6. Weng Jian-zhang. A Brief Talk on the Relationship Between Tai Ji Quan Movement and Traditional Chinese Medicine (浅谈太极拳运动与中医学的关系). *Journal of Fujian University of Traditional Chinese Medicine*. 2001, 11(2).

7. Xie Shou-de. *The Core Teachings of Tai Ji Quan Internal Practice* (太极拳内功心法). Beijing: People's Sports Publishing House; 2008.

8. Xu Bo-ran. Cultivating the Health with Wushu and its Relationship with Oriental Culture (武术养生与东方文化的关系). *China Adult Education*. 2004 (05).

9. Yang Hui. A Discussion of the Health Cultivation and Fitness Principle of Tai Ji Quan (浅谈太极拳的养生与健身原理). *Anhui Sports Technology*. 2004 (03).

10. Yang Li. *Tai Ji Quan Dictionary* (太极拳辞典). Beijing: Beijing Sport University Press; 2004.

11. Yang Ya-hong, Zhang Li-ping. A Discussion of the Health Cultivation Effect of Tai Ji Quan on the Elderly (试论太极拳对老年人的健身养生功效). *Journal of Shaoguan University*. 2004 (03).

12. Yang Zhen-duo. *Yang Style Tai Ji Quan, Sword and Blade* (杨式太极拳、剑、刀). Shanxi: Shanxi Science and Technology Press; 2002.

Index

108 *cháng quán* routine (longfist routine), 8

24 Movements Simplified Tai Ji Quan Routine, 9

32 Movements Tai Ji Sword Routine, 10

40 Movements Tai Ji Quan Competition Routine, 10

42 Movements Integrated Tai Ji Quan Routine, 10

48 Movements Tai Ji Quan Routine, 10

A

abdominal breathing, 20, 21, 37

activation effect, 14

advancing, 27

Apparent Close, 49, 77

articular cartilage, 21

ascending, 3, 12, 19

atrophy, 21

B

bā guà quán (八卦拳), 9

bā guà zhǎng, 27

basic body postures, 28

basic footwork, 29

basic hand formations, 28

Bend Bow to Shoot Tiger, 75

blood stasis, 19

body mechanics, 15

Bow Stance & Strike Groin, 71

breath regulation, 36

bump (kào, 靠), 24

C

cardio-cerebral vascular disease, 17

central equilibrium, 26

Chen Chang-xing, 7

Chen Fa-ke, 7, 9

Chen Fu-min, 6

Chen Qing-ping, 8

Chen Si-gui, 6

Chen Style Body Mechanics, 25

Chen Style Old Frame 1st Routine, 8

Chen Style Second Routine, 25

Chen style tai ji quan, 6, 24

Chen Wang-ting, 6, 7

Cheng Chang-xing, 6, 7

Chenjiagou (Chen Village), 6

Classic of the Thirty Two Forms of Fist Arts (*Quán Jīng Sān Shí Èr Shì*, 拳经三十二式), 24

Classic of the Yellow Court (*HuángTíng Jīng*, 黄庭经), 24

closing, 9, 26, 78

cold symptoms, 14

Commentary on the Classic of Changes-The Essay Series (*Yì Zhuàn-Xì Cí*, 易传-系辞), 1, 11

conscious intention (yì, 意), 15, 26

constant motion, 3

continuity, 9, 26

Cross Hands, 77

Crouch Down (Left), 69

Crouch Down (Right), 72

D

dǎo yǐn, 24

defensive effect, 14

deflect back (*lǚ*), 41

Deflect through the Back, 65

degenerative arthritis, 21

descending, 3, 12, 19

Diagonal Flying, 50

distracting thoughts, 15

Double-strike the Ears, 61

DU 20 (*bǎi huì*, 百会), 4, 28,82

DU 4 (*mìng mén*, 命门), 80

E

eight energy expressions or techniques, 24

elasticity, 25

elbow (*zhǒu*, 肘), 24

elixir field (*dān tian*, 丹田), 20, 24, 81

emission of power (*fā jìn*), 25

emptiness, 18

empty step, 12, 14, 21

entering, 3, 19

equilibrium, 3

essence-spirit, 15

exhalation, 21

exiting, 3, 19

explosive power, 9

eye of fist, 49

F

Feet Together, 33

fēng (丰), 5

fist, 28

Fist Under the Elbow, 51

flexibility, 9, 25

fluid (saliva), 20

foot stomping, 25

foot stomping force, 9

footwork, 15

force (*jìn*, 劲), 3

force (*lì*, 力), 6, 26, 44

forceful, 15

G

gaseous exchange, 20

GB 21 (*jiān jǐng*, 肩井), 30

Golden Cock Stands on One Leg, 70

Grasp the Sparrow's Tail, 40,72

H

hand techniques, 15

hands closing, 27

hands opening, 27

Hands Overlapping Posture, 29

Hands Strum the Lute, 48

Hao Wei-zhen, 7, 9, 27

hard force, 25

hardness, 6, 12, 13, 24, 25

healthy qi (*zhèng qì*), 15, 20

heart, 17

heart blood deficiency, 17

heart-shen (heart-spirit), 18

Hold the Ball Posture, 29

Hook, 28

hypertension, 18

I

inhalation, 21

initiation, 9, 26

intention (yì, 意), 6

internal practice, 6

J

jí (极), 1

jumping, 25

jumping and leaping, 25

K

KI 1 (*yǒng quán*, 涌泉), 30

L

large frame, 25

Large Frame Routine, 8

leaping, 25

Left Bow Stance, 30, 31

Left Toe Kick, 62

Li Yi-she, 7, 9

lung, 20

M

middle frame, 25

Middle Frame Routine, 8

movement, 6

N

Natural Breathing, 36

Naturalness, 35

Natural Posture, 28

navel, 29

Needle at Sea Bottom, 64

nèi jiā quán (internal wu shu), 5

new frame, 8

O

old frame, 8, 25

Opening, 30, 39

opening, 9, 26

original qi (*yuán qì*, 元气), 14

oxidative decomposition, 20

oxygen deficiency, 20

P

Palm, 28

parry (*lán*, 拦), 49

Parry & Punch, 48, 76

Part the Wild Horse's Mane (Left &Right), 56

Pat High on Horse, 60

PC 8 (*láo gōng*, 劳宫), 29

peace, 35

perineum (*huì yīn*, 会阴), 28

pluck (*cǎi*, 采), 24

post-natal, 21

power emission (*fā jìn*), 8,25

power (*jìn*), 36

pre-natal, 21

press (*jǐ*, 挤), 24, 41

Pressing Posture, 29

psychosomatic illness, 19

push (*àn*, 按), 24, 42

Q

qi (气), 6, 14, 26

Qi Ji-guang, 24

qi movement,3, 14, 17, 18, 26

qi stagnation, 19

qi transformation, 3, 17

Quan You, 7, 8

R

Raise Hands & Step Forward, 43

Ready Posture, 29, 39

regular abdominal breathing, 37

relaxation, 9, 35

retreating, 27

reverse abdominal breathing, 37

Right Bow Stance, 31, 33

Right Heel Kick, 60

Right Slap Kick, 66

S

sān (三), 5

San Feng School, 5

schools, 23

shaking, 25

shaking force, 9, 25

Single Whip, 42, 59, 72

Small Frame, 8

soft coiling movements, 25

soft power, 8

softness, 6, 12, 13, 18, 24, 25

solid step, 12, 14, 21, 27

solidity, 18

spiral-coiling (silk-reeling) energy, 25

spiral-coiling movement, 24

spiraling energy, 9

spleen, 19

split (*liè*, 挒), 24

Step Back & Straddle the Tiger, 73

Step Back & Whirl Arms, 53

Step Forward & Ward Off, 40

Step Forward to Seven Stars, 73

stillness, 6, 18

strength (*lì*), 12, 18, 24, 36

Subdue Tiger (Left & Right), 67

sudden weight shifts, 25

Sun Lu-tang, 7, 9, 27

Sun Style Body Mechanics, 27

Sun Style Tai Ji Quan, 27

T

tài (太), 1

tai ji, 1

tai ji diagram, 1, 11

Tai Ji Holism, 2

tai ji quan of opening and closing, 27

tai ji quan of opening and closingand flexible steps, 27

tailbone, 4

The Five Chen Style Old Frame Routines, 24

The Yellow Emperor's Internal Classic (*Huáng Dì Nèi Jīng*, 黄帝内经), 14, 18

tiger's mouth, 28

Treatise on Tai Ji Quan (*TàiJí Quán Lùn*, 太极拳论), 9

true qi (*zhēn qì*), 17, 21

Turn Body & Heel Kick, 63

Turn Body & Lotus Kick, 74

Turning the Body, 32

Twist Step & Brush Knee, 45

two poles, 11

U

uplifting energy (*dǐng jìn*, 顶劲), 24

upright body posture, 18, 19

V

vertex, 4

W

waist, 35

ward-off (*péng*, 掤), 24, 40, 41

warming effect, 14

Wave Hands Like Clouds, 58

Wen County, 6

White Crane Spreads Wings, 44

White Snake Spits Tongue, 65

Work Shuttle (Left & Right), 55

Wu Jian-quan, 7, 8, 26

wu shu, 1, 5, 23

Wú Style Body Mechanics, 27

Wú style tai ji quan, 8, 26

Wǔ Qín Xì (Five Animal Frolic), 5

Wǔ Style Body Mechanics, 26

Wǔ style tai ji quan, 9, 26

Wǔ Style Tai Ji Quan Competition Routine, 10

Wu Yu-xiang, 7, 9, 26

Wudang Mountain (武当山), 5

X

xíng yì quán (形意拳), 9, 27

Y

yang, 1, 11

Yang Ban-hou, 26

Yang Cheng-fu, 7, 8, 25

Yang Fu-kui, 25

Yang Jian-hou, 7, 8

Yang Lu-chan, 7, 8, 25

Yang Style body mechanics, 25

Yang style tai ji quan, 8, 25

Classic of Changes (*Yì Jīng*, 易经), 1

yield (*lǚ*, 捋), 24

yin, 1, 11

yin-yang theory, 11

Z

zang-fu (viscera and bowels), 1

Zhang San-feng (张三丰), 5,7

Zhao Bao style, 8

Zhao Bao township, 26

Zhen Wu God, 5

Zheng Man-qing, 1